Linda Bel hadj kacem
Basma Ben Barka

Risk management and biosafety

Linda Bel hadj kacem
Basma Ben Barka

Risk management and biosafety

in the pathological anatomy and cytology laboratory

ScienciaScripts

Imprint

Cover image: www.ingimage.com

This book is a translation from the original published under ISBN 978-620-6-71959-5.

Publisher:
Sciencia Scripts
is a trademark of
Dodo Books Indian Ocean Ltd. and OmniScriptum S.R.L publishing group

120 High Road, East Finchley, London, N2 9ED, United Kingdom
Str. Armeneasca 28/1, office 1, Chisinau MD-2012, Republic of Moldova, Europe
Printed at: see last page
ISBN: 978-620-8-25740-8

TABLE OF CONTENTS

INTRODUCTION

Pathological anatomy and cytology (PCA) is a medical speciality that analyses tissues and cells morphologically, using standard macroscopic, histopathological or cytological techniques. The ACP laboratory plays an essential role in the diagnosis, prognosis and monitoring of cancers and other pathological conditions (Émile et al., 2012).

However, despite technological progress and the availability of automated equipment, PCR activities rely on manual methods. Daily practices in the laboratory are characterised by the handling of infectious risk agents (fresh tissue) and the extensive use of chemicals, particularly formalin, which exposes laboratory staff to chemical, biological and physical risks at every stage of sample management (Ordre professionnel des technologistes médicaux du Québec, 2014).

Currently, the implementation of a risk management system in the PCR laboratory is a crucial procedure for improving biosafety in the laboratory, starting with the identification and understanding of hazards through to the implementation of biosafety measures that concern the health of staff and also the safety of the working environment. So how is risk management carried out? (WHO, 2006).

The aim of our work is to determine the different types of risk in the PCR laboratory at the Tunis hospital in order to implement corrective actions and preventive measures by adopting the 5M method to understand the risks and the 5S method to implement biosafety measures.

BIBLIOGRAPHICAL SUMMARY

I. LABORATORY ANATOMY AND CYTOLOGY

I.1-Definition of pathological anatomy and cytology

PCA is a medical discipline that studies morphological alterations in tissues or cells based on semiological analysis by comparing pathological tissues or cells against normal tissues in correlation with clinical data (Émile et al., 2012). The PCR examination may be an extemporaneous examination of fresh samples for rapid analysis at the time of surgery in order to obtain the opinion of the anatomical pathologist for orientation, diagnostic confirmation or an assessment of the quality of the excision in order to possibly modify the surgical procedure and guide this operation (INRS, 2013).
Histological examination is carried out on tissue fixed with formalin, dehydrated, embedded in paraffin, then cut and stained with a standard stain (haematoxylin and eosin) and analysed by microscopic observation (INRS, 2013).
Cytological samples are spread on slides, fixed with alcohol and stained with various special stains (Papanicolaou, Giemsa, Ziehl Nelson, Rouge Congo, etc.) depending on the nature of the cells (Émile et al., 2012).

I.2- Role and missions of the laboratory

The PCR laboratory has three main roles:

- Diagnosis: this involves analysing lesions and describing the morphology of tissue or cytological samples by macroscopic and microscopic examination in order to confirm a diagnosis or propose a diagnostic hypothesis (Émile et al., 2012) (INRS, 2013).
- Prognosis: this role is linked to tumour pathologies by determining the main prognostic factors such as infiltration, grade, pTNM stage and lymph node dissection (Émile et al., 2012).
- Evaluate a therapeutic approach: determine an effective targeted therapy by studying theranostic factors (Her2neu, hormone receptors, etc.) such as the expression of tumour markers (Émile et al, 2012).

I.3- Management of pathological anatomy and cytology samples :

On arrival at the laboratory, the sample goes through various stages until the histological or cytological result is validated. Fixation: immediately after sampling, the sample must be fixed in 10% buffered formalin to fix the tissue and prevent cell autolysis.

Macroscopic study: this stage is carried out by a pathologist. It consists of a macroscopic examination (size, colour and appearance) of the sample and its dissection using a scalpel to form cassettes.
For rigid samples (bone or cartilage), the sample must be decalcified using an acid. Automated Circulation: the tissue must be treated to eliminate free water. This stage is generally automated, with the tissue passing through various chemicals such as formalin,

alcohol and xylene in order to fix it better, dehydrate it and finally impregnate it with a small quantity of liquid paraffin.

Paraffin embedding: once the tissue has been dehydrated, it is embedded in liquid paraffin to form a support in the form of a paraffin block.

Microtomy: using a microtome fitted with a sharp blade, 3μm tissue sections are cut manually and placed on slides in a water bath.

Standard haematoxylin and eosin (HE) stain: this is a routine stain which highlights the nucleus and tissue structures.

Mounting the slides: once the slides have been stained, they are covered with a coverslip using the Eukitt.

Reading the results: the slides are read under an optical microscope by a pathologist to establish a diagnosis.

Report writing: the PCR report includes the results of the macroscopic and microscopic examinations and any additional analyses.

Storage: the spare part must be stored in appropriate packaging and in ventilated cupboards.

To ensure the integrity of paraffin slides and blocks, they must be filed and stored under appropriate conditions with the correct temperature and humidity (Ordre professionnel des technologistes médicaux du Québec, 2014).

Waste disposal**:** waste produced in the ACP must be sorted and classified. in :

- Waste similar to household waste.
- Waste from high-risk healthcare activities

Household and similar waste is collected in black bags and disposed of by municipal services, with the main option of disposal in controlled landfill sites. Hazardous waste must be disposed of through a specific channel.
This second category of waste must itself be divided into :

- Toxic or chemical waste
- Anatomical or infectious risk waste
- Sharp waste

Each category of hazardous waste must be disposed of through a specific channel.

Chemical waste, mainly used solvents and acids, is collected in red bags and reactive products should not be mixed (e.g., solvents, acids, etc.).

The more the waste is mixed, the more expensive it will be to destroy. Finally, the waste is sent to an authorised disposal centre and undergoes a physical-chemical treatment.

Infectious risk waste must be collected in yellow bags before disposal (ANGED, 2012).

Anatomical parts are disposed of by burial.

Sharps waste must be collected in solid plastic regie boxes and disposed of by specialist companies.This hazardous waste must be disposed of through a specific channel (Ordre professionnel des technologistes médicaux du Québec, 2014).

II. THE DIFFERENT RISKS AT A ANATOMY AND PATHOLOGICAL CYTOLOGY LABORATORY

II.1-Definition of risk

According to ISO 31000, a risk is an effect of the uncertainty of objectives, generally expressed in terms of risk source, events and their consequences (ISO.org,a). The WHO defines risk as the probability or possibility of an undesirable event causing harm (WHO, 2006).

II.1.a-Chemical risks

Chemical risks in the PCR laboratory concern all the chemical substances commonly used in the day-to-day practice of pathology and which cause short- and long-term harmful effects to exposed professionals (Costa et al., 2008).

Figure 1: Chemical hazard logo (INRS, 2013)

II.1.a.1-Formol

Formaldehyde is an organic compound belonging to the aldehyde family. It is traditionally used as a tissue fixative in the PCR laboratory due to its low cost and effective preservation (Costa et al., 2008).

The International Agency for Research on Cancer (IARC) has classified formalin as a carcinogen, and it is a potential factor in the development of nasopharyngeal cancer and myeloid leukaemia. Studies have shown the toxic effect of exposure to formalin, it causes skin irritations such as dermatitis and eye irritations as well as other respiratory problems such as asthma (Joshi et al., 2017).

It also causes headaches, neurotoxicity, chromosomal aberrations and DNA damage.

For pregnant women, it can cause congenital degeneration of the foetus. The frequency of exposure to formalin differs according to the activity of the staff, with the areas where samples are dissected having the highest level ofexposure, approximately 0.6 and 1.3 ppm (d'Ettorre et al., 2017). The exposure limit for formalin is 0.3 ppm over 8 hours (d'Ettorre et al., 2017).

II.1.a.2- Xylene

It is a chemical compound belonging to the family of aromatic hydrocarbons used in the ACP laboratory in the treatment of tissues with the 'technicon' automaton, colouring and editing (Andrion and Pira, 1994). It is a highly flammable product harmful by inhalation, skin and eye contact (Joshi et al, 2017). Short- and long-term exposure causes nausea, dizziness, vomiting, anorexia and abdominal pain, as well as excitation, drowsiness, central nervous system depression and respiratory disorders (Joshi et al., 2017).

II.1.a.3-Alcohol

Organic compound belonging to the hydroxyl group used in the PCR laboratory to hydrate and dehydrate tissues, also used as a fixative in cytology (INRS, 2013).
Chronic exposure to high doses of alcohol causes dry skin and irritant dermatitis (INRS, 2013).

II.1.a.4-Colouring products

The dyes used in ACP are aromatic amines, which are toxic depending on the concentration of each substance and the exposure time for each dye (INRS, 2013). Some dyes, such as eosin, are non-toxic, but others, such as Congo Red and Fushin, are considered carcinogenic by accumulation. The mercury monoxide used in Harris haematoxylin is highly toxic (INRS, 2013).

II.1.a.5-Decalcifying solutions

Decalcification products are commonly used in the PCR laboratory on bone and cartilage samples, this makes microtome cutting easier (INRS, 2013). The most commonly used decalcifiers include nitric acid, acetic acid, ferric acid and hydrochloric acid. Acids all have corrosive properties that cause severe mucocutaneous lesions and eye damage. serious.In addition, these products are highly flammable and combustible, and some of the acids are toxic, mutagenic and sensitising (INRS, 2013).

II.2.b- Physical risks

In the PCR laboratory, staff are exposed to various types of physical hazards such as injuries, fire hazards, equipment hazards and musculoskeletal and vision disorders (Andrion and Pira, 1994).

Figure 2: Logo for a physical risk (INRS, 2013)

II.2.b.1-Injury

Injuries are common in the PCR laboratory, and studies have shown that cuts, lacerations from sharp tools and needle sticks are a common hazard in pathology practice. Indeed, macroscopy is the riskiest activity, with 82% of pathologists reporting at least one injury in their career in specimen dissection where hands are most exposed (Fritzsche et al., 2012). Technicians are also exposed to the risk of injury when changing the sharp blades of the microtome, but this risk is less frequent (Adyanthaya and Jose, 2013).

II.2.b.2-Fire

The risk of fire in the PCR laboratory is associated with the use of several combustible and flammable chemicals as well as equipment that presents a source of heat and a source of sparks (INRS, 2013). Paraffin is a combustible material that increases the risk of fire in the presence of a flammable source. Formaldehyde, toluene, xylene and ethanol are highly flammable at temperatures above 37°C. The presence of these products with a source of spark or heat is sufficient to cause a fire (Adyanthaya and Jose, 2013).

I.2.b.3-Electrical shock

The risk of electric shock is related to equipment and PLCs used in the PCR laboratory that are electrically live can cause electrical problems such as current leakage (Joshi et al., 2017).

II.2.b.4-Ergonomic problems

II.2.b.4.1- Musculoskeletal disorders

These disorders are associated with the use of the microscope by pathologists; in fact, one study showed that 3/4 of Swiss pathologists suffer from musculoskeletal problems in the neck and shoulders (Fritzsche et al., 2012).

II.2.b.4.2- Vision problems

Visual problems are very common among PCR laboratory staff, with 89% of pathologists using the microscope suffering from myopia (Fritzsche et al., 2012).

II.2.c-Biological risks

Biological risks in the PCR laboratory mainly concern fresh unfixed samples, since fixed tissue does not present a biological risk since the fixative deactivates the micro-organisms (Andrion and Pira, 1994). Extemporaneous examination is the riskiest activity, since staff are exposed to unfixed tissue or other biological fluids through contact or inhalation. Biological risk also exists during the reception and disposal of fresh tissues (Andrion and Pira, 1994).

Figure 3: Biohazard logo (INRS, 2013)

The most common transmissible infectious agents in the PCR laboratory are : Tuberculosis: Tuberculosis contamination is a potential risk for pathologists and technicians, particularly those working in cytology and cytopuncture as well as extemporaneous examination, contamination occurs through contact when dissecting fresh tissue or handling cytological fluid (Adyanthaya and Jose, 2013).

Hepatitis B: Hepatitis B infection is also known to be a risk for ACP workers, with sharp tool wounds and eye droplets being the main routes of contamination (Adyanthaya and Jose, 2013). HIV: This is a virus that can be accidentally transmitted to staff during the handling of fresh tissues or other infected biological fluids, through mucocutaneous contact, but the risk of contamination is low at around 0.3% (Adyanthaya and Jose, 2013).

III. MANAGEMENT OF RISKS AT A ANATOMY AND PATHOLOGICAL CYTOLOGY LABORATORY

III.1 ISO 31000 standard: Risk management

The ISO 31000 standard, developed by the ISO/TC262 technical committee, is a set of guidelines to help organisations effectively identify and mitigate risk. ISO 31000 was developed in 2 editions, the first in 2009 and the 2nd in 2018, which is more strategic and emphasises the involvement of management in risk management within the organisation (iso.org,a).

III.1.a-Definition of risk management

According to ISO 31000, it is the set of activities coordinated in a well-defined process that enables risks to be identified and assessed with the aim of controlling and minimising any risk that has occurred (iso.org,a).

III.1.b-Objective of the ISO 31000 standard

The ISO 31000 standard enables organisations and employees to develop a risk management culture and strengthen their knowledge of risk management. This standard helps to put in place a risk management system and strategy that helps to respond effectively and rapidly to a risk (iso.org,a).

III.1.c-Principles of the ISO31000 standard

ISO 31000 is based on 8 principles:

1- Integrated: risk management is part of the organisation's activities and management's responsibility.

2- Structured and comprehensive: risk management must be structured with a guideline and all staff must be involved.

3- Adapted: risk management is not a one-size-fits-all approach; it must be adapted to the organisation's activities, objectives and environment.

4- Inclusive: all stakeholders must be included in the risk management process.

5- Dynamic: risk management must be responsive to change and anticipatory.

6- Best available information: all information must be known and made available.

7- Human and cultural factors: risk management is influenced by human behaviour.

8- Continuous improvement: risk management encourages continuous improvement. (iso.org,a)

III.1.d-Risk management processes

Identifying risks: describing events, risks, sources, causes and consequences. Analyse the risks: determine the nature of the risk, the level of exposure, the probability and the possible scenarios.Assess the risks: compare the results of the analysis with the risk criteria and determine the necessary measures. Dealing with risks: drawing up and implementing an action plan. (iso.org,a)

III.2-5M method

The 5M method, also known as the Ishikawa diagram, is a method developed in 1962 by the Japanese engineer and quality control expert Kaoru Ishikawa. It is a tool for studying the causes and effects of a problem (Geradus, 2020).The structure of the diagram resembles the skeleton of a fish, with the ribs representing the causes ofa problem and the head showing the effect (Geradus, 2020).This diagram structures the causes of a problem in 5M, which are :

- Environment: workstation and surroundings.
- Method: work procedures and techniques.
- Workforce: staff in terms of qualifications and skills.
- Materials: work equipment.
- Material: the material used in the workstation.

The 5M method is useful in risk management, enabling a detailed assessment of a probable risk (Harzli, 2021).

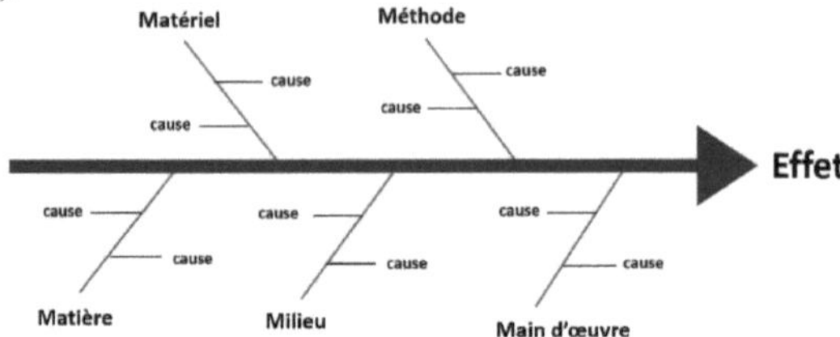

Figure 4: Structure of the Ishikawa diagram modified from (Geradus, 2020)

IV. BIOSECURITY IN AN ANATOMY AND PATHOLOGY LABORATORY

IV.1-Definition

According to ISO 35001, it is the set of practices and controls designed to reduce the risk of exposure or unintentional release of a biological or other material used in the laboratory (Iso.org,b).

According to the WHO, biosafety in a laboratory is the set of containment principles and practices that prevent involuntary exposure to pathogenic or toxic agents or their accidental release (WHO, 2006).

IV.2-Principle

Biosafety is based on the presence of the following personnel and environmental protection elements: Personal protection measures: laboratory staff must wear protective equipment appropriate to their role in the laboratory (WHO, 2006). Collective protection measures: the laboratory must be equipped with equipment and materials that ensure the safety of the environment (WHO, 2006).

IV.3-Objective

Biosafety enables :

✓Ensuring the health and safety of laboratory staff.

✓Ensuring environmental safety in the laboratory.

✓Minimising exposure to risks in the laboratory.

✓Improved working conditions and productivity in the laboratory. (WHO, 2006)

IV.4 - ISO 35001 standard: Laboratory biohazard management system

The ISO 35001 standard, published in December 2019, is based on occupational health and safety management standards and focuses on the specific nature of biohazard management in laboratories (ISO.org,b). This standard represents the process and framework for effective biosafety management, ensuring the safety of personnel and guaranteeing the reliability of results. The biohazard management system is based on the process of identifying, assessing, controlling and managing biological or other risks associated with the laboratory (ISO.org,b).

IV.5-5S method

IV.5.a-General description of the method

The 5S method is a Japanese method developed by Tahich Ohno in 1991 on Toyota production sites (ASQ, 2009).It is a method of organising the workplace, providing a clean, well-organised and safe working environment to reduce waste and optimise productivity (ASQ, 2009). 5S comes from the following 5 Japanese words:

Table I: The 5 actions of the 5S method

Japanese words	Translation	French word	Explanation
Seiri	Eliminate	Delete	Separate the necessary tools from the unnecessary ones. deleted
Seiton	Ranger	Visit	Organise, order and file tools and equipment The materials for facilitate their use
Seiso	Clean	Scintillate	Cleaning the workspace and keeping equipment clean and well-maintained
Seiketsu	Standardise	Standardise	Establishing and planning rules to be followed daily
Shituke	Respect	Follow	Follow and respect the first 4 S

A 6th S can be added, "Safety", but this is not a sequential step, it must be considered throughout the 5S presented in the following figure. Safety must be both a means and an end of the 5S (ASQ, 2009).

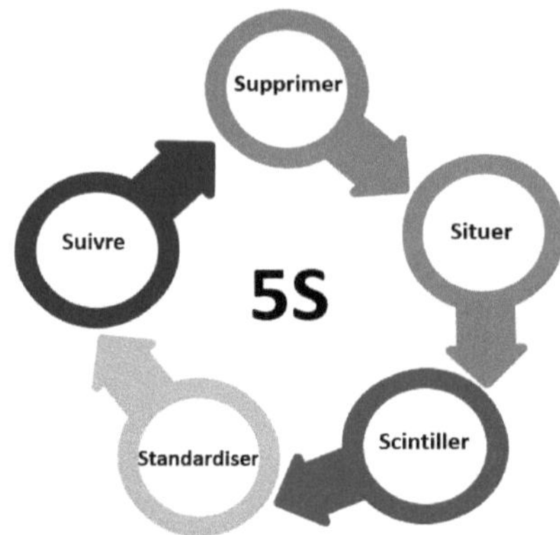

Figure 5: The 5 actions of the 5S method (ASQ, 2009)

IV.5.b-Application of 5S in the PCR laboratory

The 5S method can be applied to any workspace, including the PCR laboratory, a workplace that requires a method for organising it. Applying this method in the PCR laboratory improves the quality of work through better availability of equipment and a clean, well-organised workspace, which increases productivity (ASQ, 2009). This method is important in terms of safety by reducing sources of risk and offers more comfortable working conditions (Drillaud et al., 2016).

IV.6-Prevention measures in the PCR laboratory

Several types of risk have been identified in the PCR laboratory, which means that a biosafety system needs to be put in place to minimise the risks through various individual, collective and organisational recommendations (INRS, 2013).

Personal protection measures: to protect the health of each employee, these measures include personal protective equipment such as a waterproof overblouse, disposable sleeve, goggles or visor, gloves adapted to each activity (latex, nitrile, cut-resistant), overshoes, calluses, mask (surgical, FFP2, chemical filter) as well as personal hygiene, essentially washing hands before and after each activity (Lisa, 2017).

Medical surveillance has been recommended including vaccination (Adyanthaya and Jose, 2013). Collective protection measures: to protect the environment and all personnel. These measures are essentially the presence of a ventilation system to reduce the risk of exposure to chemical agents by inhalation, as well as the presence of a chemical extraction hood, a microbiological safety cabinet and ventilated cupboards for storing samples (Lisa, 2017). The upkeep and preventive maintenance of equipment are almost essential for the safety of personnel against electricity-related risks (Adyanthaya and Jose, 2013). Regular staff training must be incorporated into the laboratory's activity plan, to ensure that the work team is aware of the various possible risks in the laboratory, to guarantee compliance with safety practices and adaptation to recommendations, as well as the implementation of corrective actions and management in the event of exposure to the various risks (Adyanthaya and Jose, 2013). Installing earth leakage circuit breakers (ELCBs) protects equipment and, consequently, personnel. In the event of an electricity leak, the circuit breakers automatically cut off the current (Adyanthaya and Jose, 2013).

Organisational preventive measures: These measures protect employees and the environment at the same time.
The recommendations mainly concern the architecture of the laboratory:

-Activities must be separated at different locations (INRS, 2013).

-Access must be restricted to department staff (INRS, 2013).

-Chemicals must be stored in appropriate premises, respecting the storage temperature (INRS, 2013).
-Each chemical product must be labelled with its name, hazard warnings and safety procedures (INRS, 2013).
-Separate chemical products from flammable products or automatic machines that can be a source of heat (INRS, 2013).
The presence of signs in the laboratory is recommended; these signs include prohibited activities (drinking, eating, smoking) and biosafety recommendations (individual prevention measures) (INRS, 2013).

Waste sorting is a vital step in minimising risks, so ordinary waste must be separated from waste that poses a chemical, biological or physical risk (INRS, 2013).

STUDY OBJECTIVE

The aim of our work is :

- ►Identifying possible risks in the PCR laboratory
- ►Evaluate biosafety measures in the laboratory
- ►Implement corrective and preventive actions

MATERIALS AND METHODS

I. MATERIAL

I.1-Inclusion criteria

Our study takes into account all activities within the PCR laboratory at the hospital in Tunis and all staff working during the period from February to May 2023.

I.2-Exclusion criteria

Our study excludes the risks associated with the molecular biology unit, since this is a limited activity, not specific to the PCR laboratory.
We have also excluded non-permanent staff.

I.3-Premises and staff

I-3-a-Personnel :

The staff of the laboratory are distributed as follows:

- 5 doctors and 6 residents
- 7 technicians
- 3 secretaries
- 3 researchers
- 2 receptionists
- A worker

The staff organisation chart is shown in the figure below

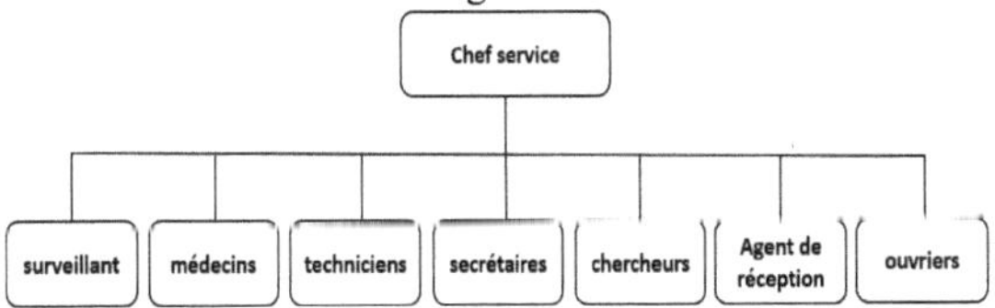

Figure 6: Laboratory staff organisation chart

I.3.b- Premises: architecture

The ACP laboratory is made up of technical units and administrative office units, as illustrated in the figure below:

- Reception room: n°1
- Macroscopy room: n°2
- Technical room: n°3
- Colouring room: n°4
- Doctors' offices: n°10, 14, 18, 19
- Staff room: n°12
- Cytopuncture room: n°13
- Secretarial office: n°11
- Supervisor's office: no. 5
- Head of department's office: n°15
- Immunohistochemistry room: n°6
- Molecular biology room: n°8,9
- Archive room: n°16
- Cloakroom: n°7
- Toilet block: n°17

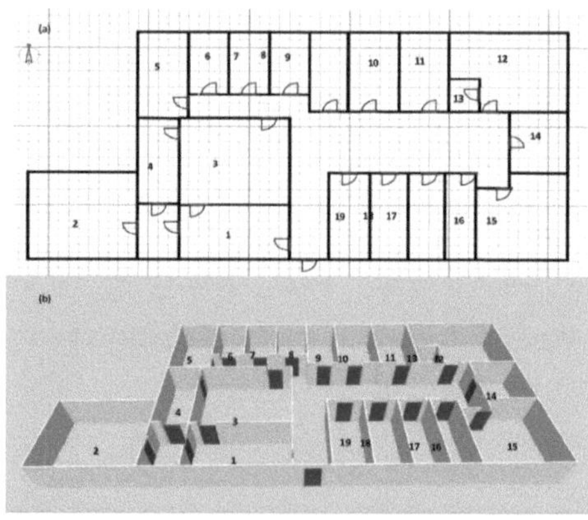

Figure 7: Plan of the laboratory (a) top view, (b) 3D view

I.4-Laboratory equipment

I.4.a-Samples

All histological samples (biopsies, surgical specimens and autopsies) and cytological samples (punctures and smears) handled in the laboratory.

I.4.b-Equipment and material

All the laboratory equipment: fume hood, automated inclusion system, automated circulation system, dissection equipment (scalpel), microtome, microscope, slides and coverslips.

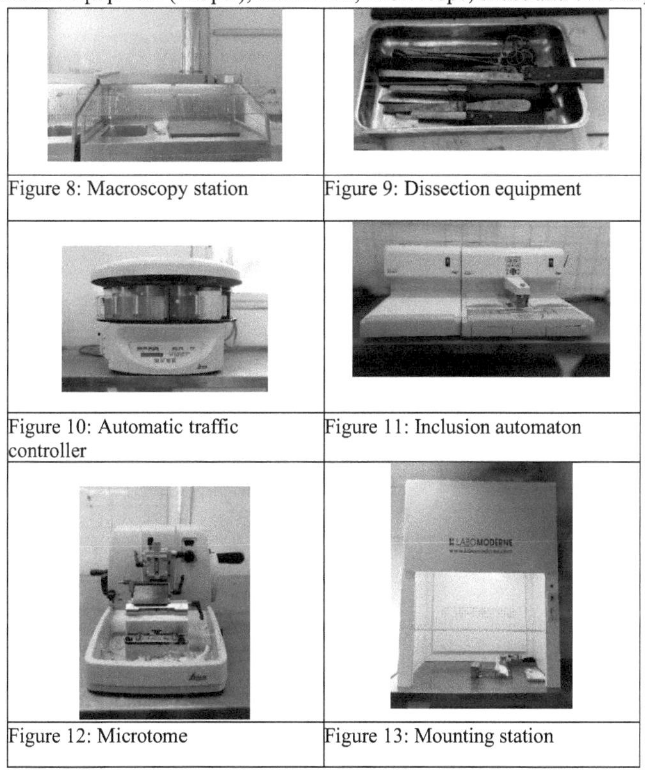

Figure 8: Macroscopy station

Figure 9: Dissection equipment

Figure 10: Automatic traffic controller

Figure 11: Inclusion automaton

Figure 12: Microtome

Figure 13: Mounting station

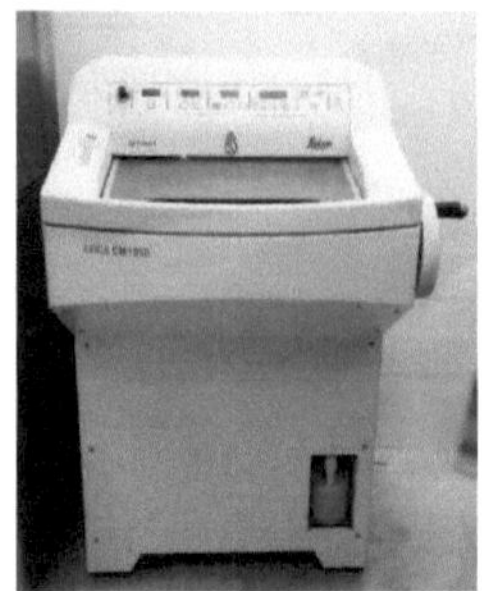

Figure 14: Cryostat automated extemporaneous examination system

I.4.c- Products and reagents

Products used in tissue treatment, including fixatives (formalin), xylene, alcohol, dyes, decalcifier and Eukitt.

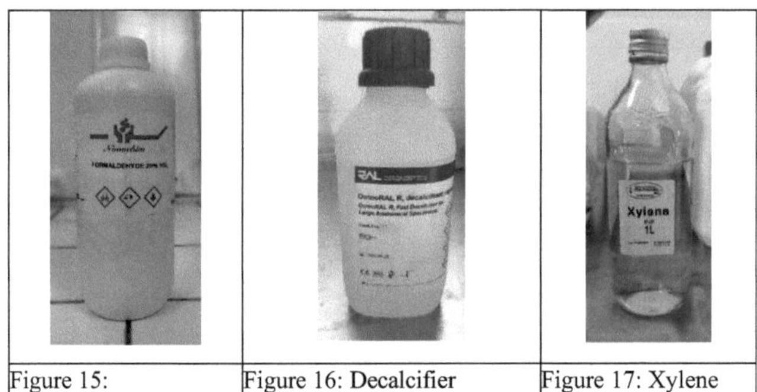

Figure 15: Formaldehyde	Figure 16: Decalcifier	Figure 17: Xylene

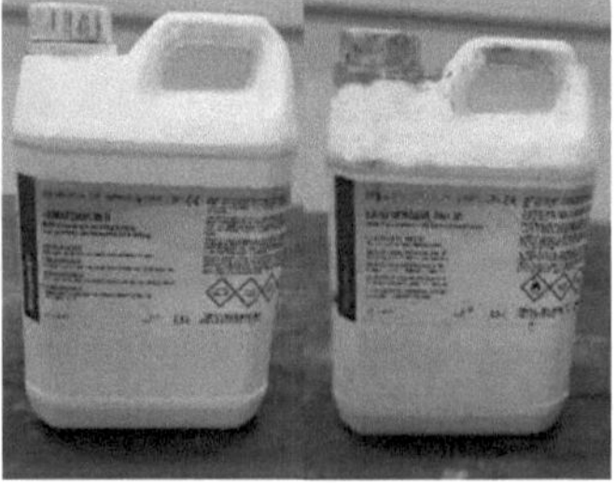

Figure 18: Dyes

II.METHODS

II.1-Presentation of the study

This is a descriptive, observational and prospective study of the PCR laboratory at the Tunis hospital, including all staff, premises, equipment and materials, as well as samples, over the period February to May 2023.Risk management is carried out in accordance with the ISO 31000 risk management process, using the 5M method to study risks and their impact on the company. 5S method for implementing biosafety measures.

II.2- ISO 31000 risk management process

For risk management in the laboratory, we have followed the ISO 31000 process through the following stages:

1- Identifying risks: during the work placement we observed and described the different types of risk that are possible in the laboratory.
2- Analyse the risks: we classified the risks into 3 types (chemical, physical, biological) and then determined the risks associated with each activity. 3-Assess risks and biosafety measures: we determined
the probability of occurrence of a risk and the presence or absence of biosafety measures.
4- Dealing with risks: we have put in place corrective actions and biosafety measures.

II.3-5M method: risk management

To study the causes of the risks, we applied the Ishikawa diagram, illustrated in the figure below.Risks are broken down into the following 5Ms: Materials: all the laboratory's equipment (technical equipment, automatic machines, IT equipment) and the reagents used. Material: samples analysed (histological and cytological). Method: operating procedure. Workforce: laboratory staff (doctors, technicians, secretaries).Environment: the environment, the different premises and the laboratory units.

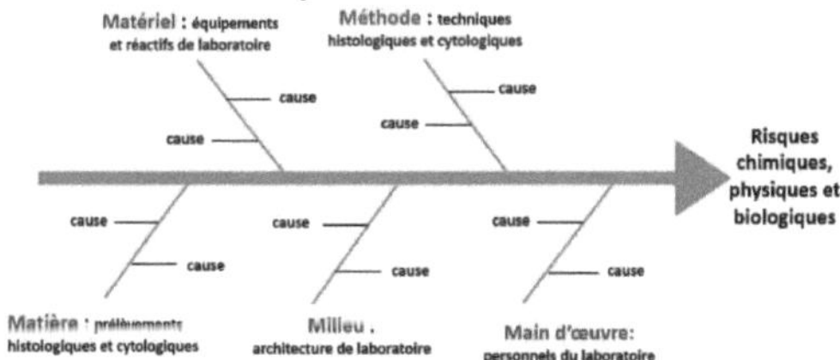

Figure 19: Ishikawa diagram

II.4- 5S method: Biosafety

To improve biosafety measures, we applied the 5S method in the laboratory, in line with its philosophy. Our method is aimed at the entire PCR laboratory and involves all staff.

1- Eliminate: we have sorted the objects in the laboratory and eliminated those that are no longer needed. This involves sorting waste (ordinary waste, biological and chemical waste) to avoid cluttering the bench and prevent chemical and biological risks.

2- Situate: we have arranged the different work areas, separated the storage area for chemical, biological, office automation and documentation products and arranged the equipment according to its use.
3- Scintillation: the premises and workbenches are cleaned daily, which involves decontaminating the materials used in extemporaneous examinations.
4- Standardising: we have put up posters identifying the different types of risk and the preventive measures to be followed, as well as good practice. We also prepared and distributed brochures to staff to raise awareness and inform them about the risks, how to deal with exposure and prevention measures (see appendix).
5- Monitoring: we checked that biosafety measures were respected in the laboratory to ensure that this method was applied.

II.5-Questionnaire

To assess knowledge and determine the different types of risk for the various laboratory staff, we drew up a questionnaire for all staff in the PCR laboratory at the hospital in Tunis. The questionnaire was printed in 2 pages (see appendix) containing 13 questions that are the same for all staff.

RESULTS

I. DENTIFICATION AND CLASSIFICATION OF RISKS

During the training period we noted the presence of different types of risk during the various stages of sample management:

I.1- Acceptance :

The receptionist was exposed to :

• Chemical risks through inhalation and skin contact: poorly sealed containers and sheets soiled with formaldehyde.
• Biological risks from contact with a fresh sample intended for an extemporaneous examination which is not properly packaged and from sheets soiled with blood or other biological fluids.
A receptionist was contaminated and contracted pulmonary tuberculosis, which was treated with anti-tuberculosis drugs for 6 months.
The following figures show the sources of risk in the reception area.

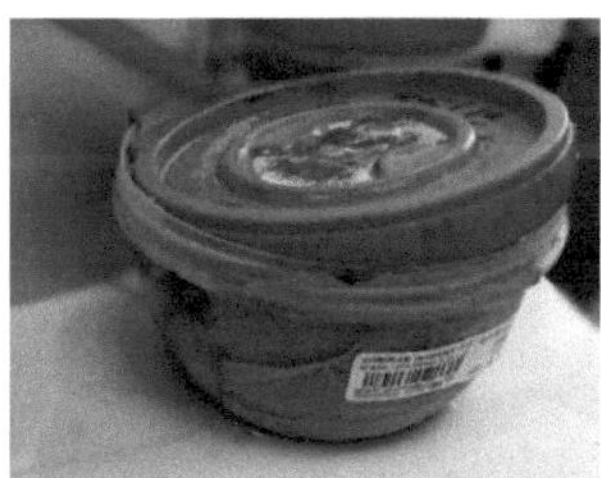

Figure 20: A poorly closed container (cap not fitting the bottle)

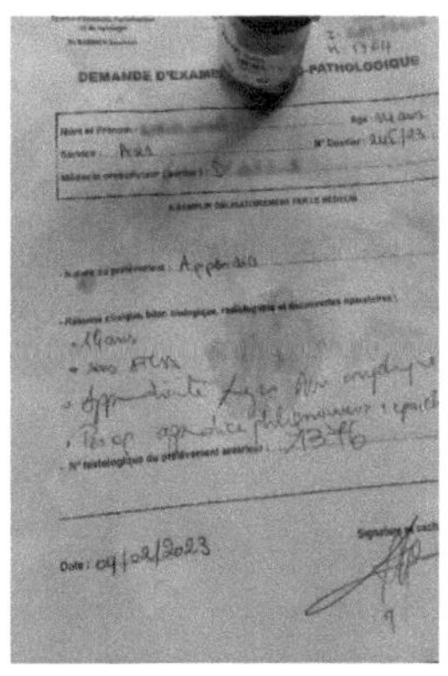

Figure 21: Formalin-stained leaf

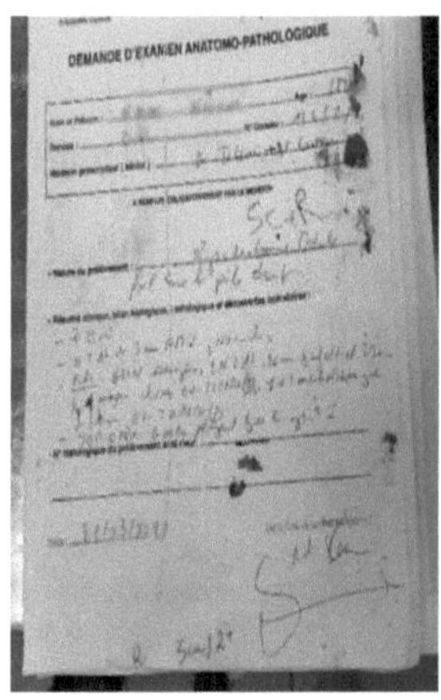

DEMANDE D'EXAMEN ANATOMO-PATHOLOGIQUE

Figure 22: Request form for an examination soiled with blood

I.2- Macroscopic stage :

This activity presented the 3 types of risk.

The sample handler in the macroscopy room was exposed to chemicals through :

- Inhalation, especially of fixative vapours during tissue dissection fixed.
- Mucocutaneous contact during the preparation of formalin and during the decalcification of tissue using acids.
- Ocular route by accidental projection

Incidents of injury were recorded, one case of a deep wound in a resident who required sutures, but the other cases of injury were superficial and minor.
The following figures show the risks associated with the macroscopy bench.

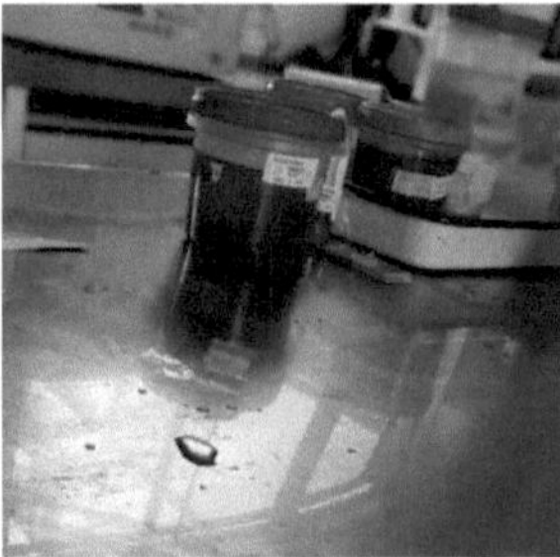

Figure 23: Drop of formalin on the macroscopy bench

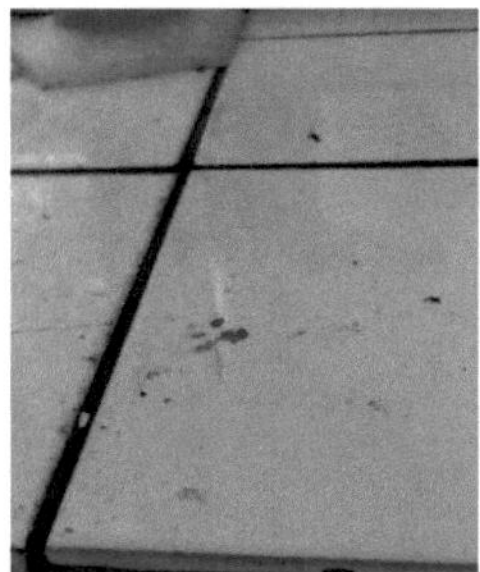

Figure 24: Blood-stained bench in the macroscopy room

I.3- Extemporaneous examination

Doctors handling fresh tissue were exposed to blood through mucocutaneous contact. No cases of contamination by infectious agents were recorded.

I.4- Traffic :

This stage is automated, and the risk existed when the solvents, mainly xylene and formaldehyde, were refilled in the automat, where staff were exposed to the vapours of toxic chemicals.

I.5- Paraffin embedding :

No incidents of liquid paraffin burns were recorded, nor were any incidents of electricity leaks or electric shocks.

I.6- Microtomy :

Each week, at least one case of injury was noted among the technicians during the changing of microtome blades. The figure below shows a microtome and slides.

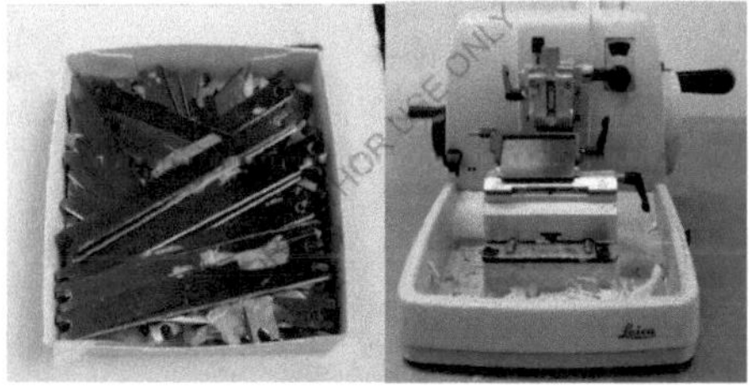

Figure 25: Cutting blades and microtome

I.7- Staining :

Staining in our laboratory is purely manual (preparation of stains and handling of slides). The operator was exposed to the staining products through the skin and by inhaling the vapours released when handling the slides and staining baths (figure 26).

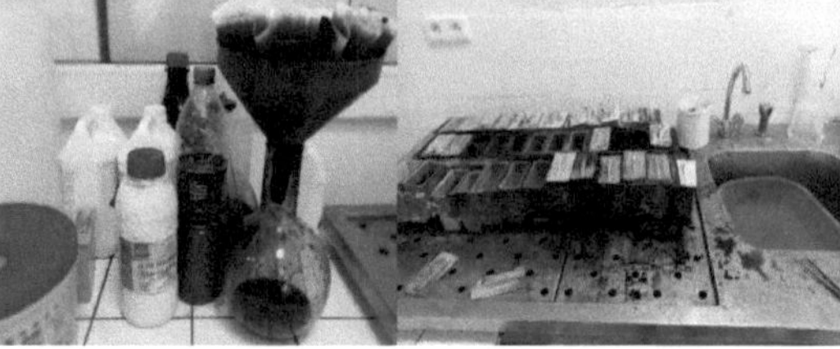

Figure 26: Staining bench

I.8- Assembly :

The operator was exposed to inhalation of xylene and Eukitt vapours and to skin contact from splashes when mounting the slides (Figure 27).

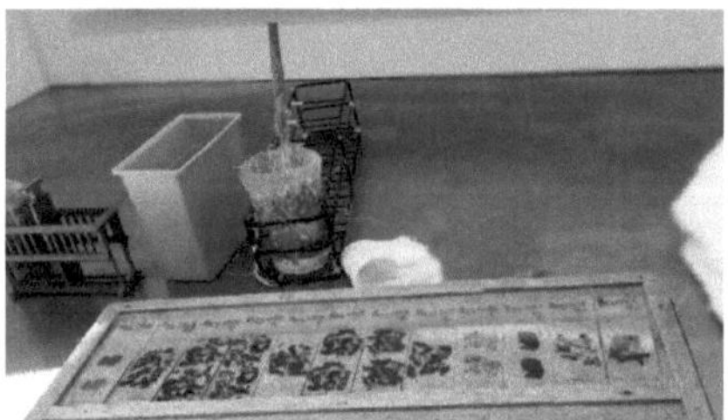

Figure 27: Fitting the blades

I.9- Reading slides :

This stage was less risky in terms of chemical risks, but was characterised by the presence of ergonomic problems, in particular musculoskeletal problems and visual problems.
Doctors were also exposed to infectious risks when searching for microcrystals in joint fluids.

I.10- Entering the report :

Chemical and biological risks were present through skin contact with the examination request sheet soiled with blood or formalin.

I.11- Waste storage and disposal :

Storage of reserves :Once the macroscopic examination has been carried out, the rest of the anatomical parts are stored. During the period February and March 2023, reserve storage did not comply with regulations. We noted the presence of reserves in This is illustrated in the figure below.

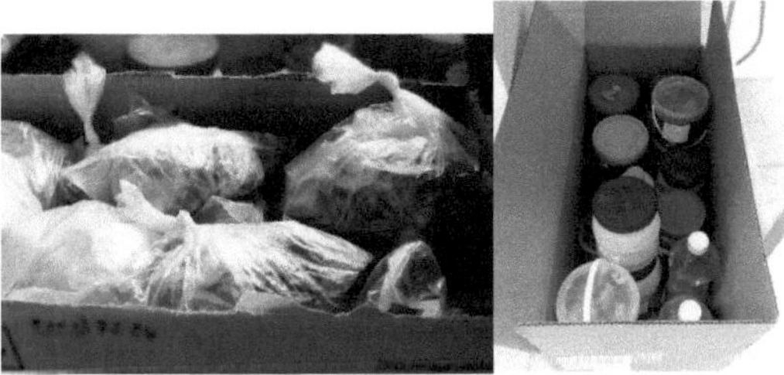

Figure 28: Storage of reserves in fragile bags and cardboard boxes

By April 2023, reserve storage conditions had been improved (inventilated cupboards).

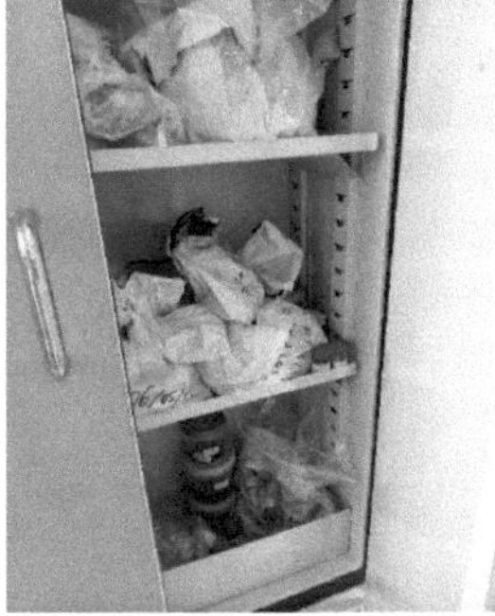

Figure 29: Reserves in a ventilated cabinet

Blade and block storage :

Although there are binders of boards and blocks, the problem is where the binders are stored. We observed boards and blocks filed in binders and stored in the corridors and in the toilet block. We also noted the presence of broken blades on a daily basis, as shown in the figure below.

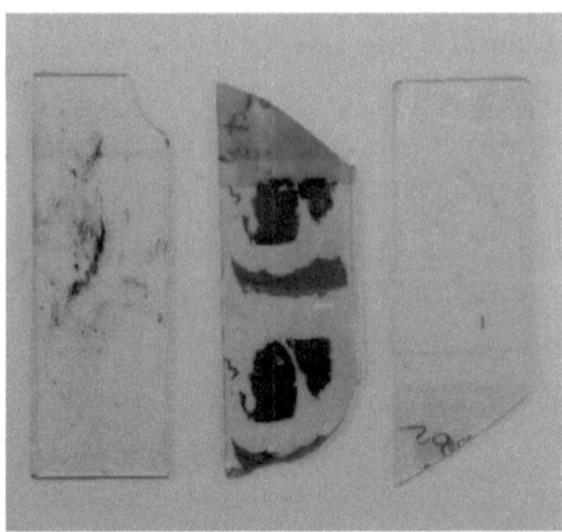

Figure 30: Broken blades (sharp elements)

Storage of chemicals :

The chemicals were stored as follows in suitable cabinets, in compliance with storage conditions (Figure 31).

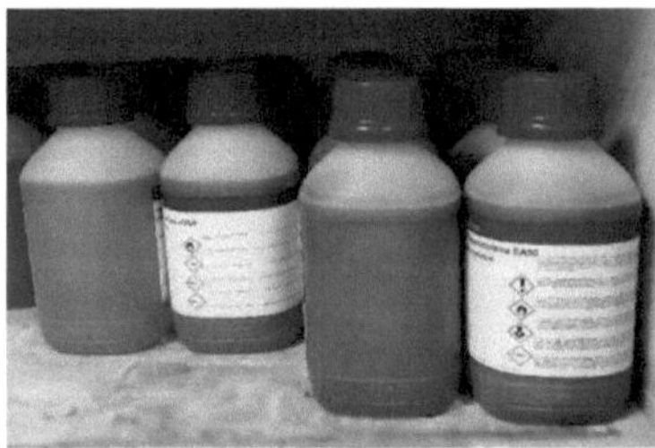

Figure 31: Chemical storage

The problem with chemical products is that they are displaced during daily use. We have noted the presence of products chemicals flammable on the same bench as shown in the figure below.

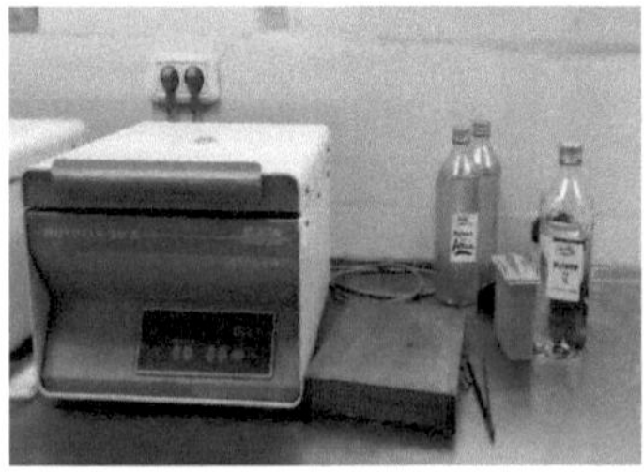

Figure 32: Bottle of xylene next to a centrifuge (risk of explosion)

Waste disposal :

Staff were exposed to infectious and chemical risks through contact with chemical and blood-stained waste. We noted a lack of compliance with waste sorting rules, despite the presence of different types of bags for chemical and infectious risks, as illustrated in the figure below.

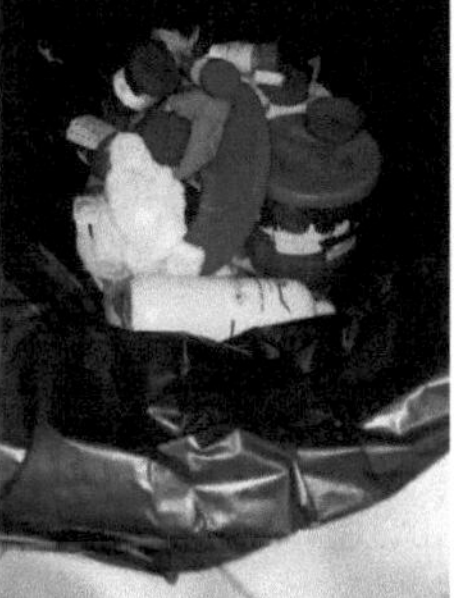

Figure 33: Chemical and biological waste in a black bag for household waste

- The study of the causes of the risks was assessed using the 5M method

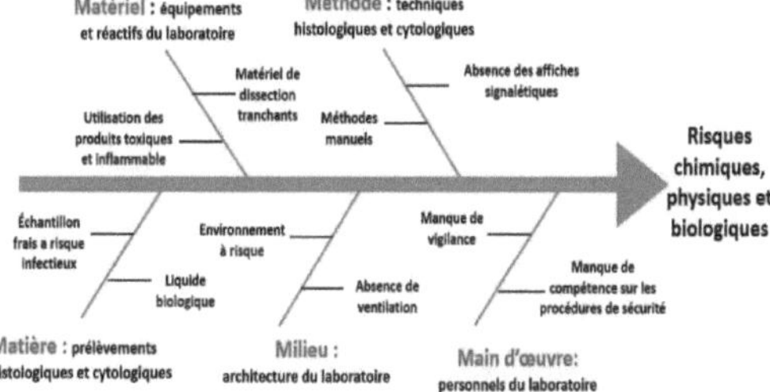

Figure 34: Presentation of risk causes using the Ishikawa diagram

II- BIOSAFETY MEASURES

During the training period we noted the availability of the following protective measures:

II.1- Individual protection measures

The personal protective equipment available was : Gloves (nitrile), overblouse (disposable and waterproof), masks (surgical, FFP2, chemical filtration), goggles and visor. The chemical filtration mask used in the laboratory is shown in the figure below. The gloves available were size L; sizes S and M were not available The use of this personal protective equipment was not observed by all staff. We noted that receptionists did not use gloves. The chemical filtration mask was used only by a few doctors in the macroscopy room, and no female technician wore this type of mask in the macroscopy room. We noted the absence of cut-resistant gloves in the department.

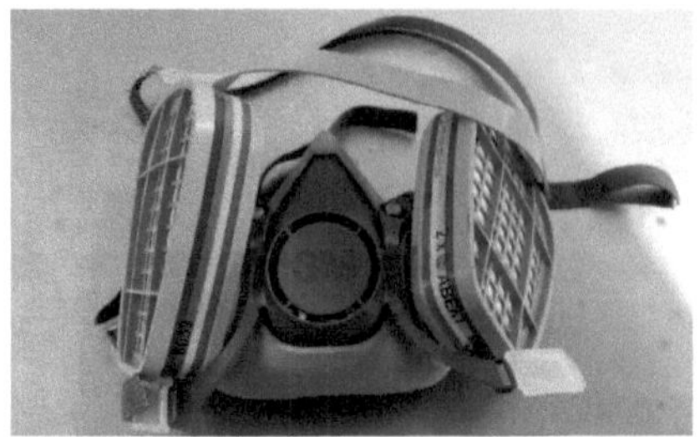

Figure 35: Chemical filtration mask

II.2- Collective protection measures

The ventilation system was absent until the beginning of April 2023.This problem was resolved following the installation of a ventilation system (figure 36) in April 2023 and the installation of a chemical extraction hood (figure 39) in the blade assembly room. The macroscopy room was equipped with ventilated cupboards (Figure 37) for the storage of supplies, as well as a washbasin and an eye-wash fountain (Figure 38).

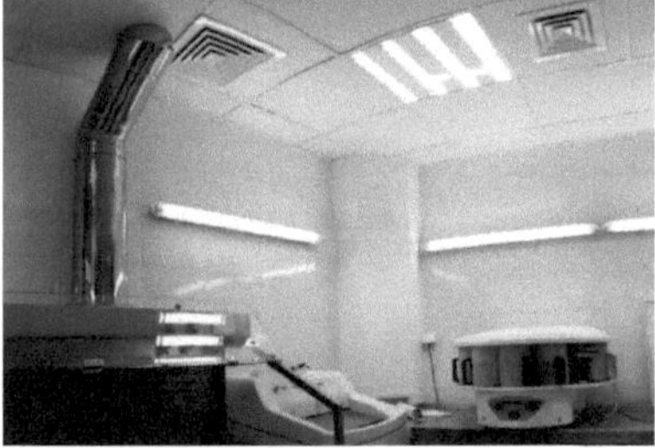

Figure 36: Ventilation system in the macroscopy room

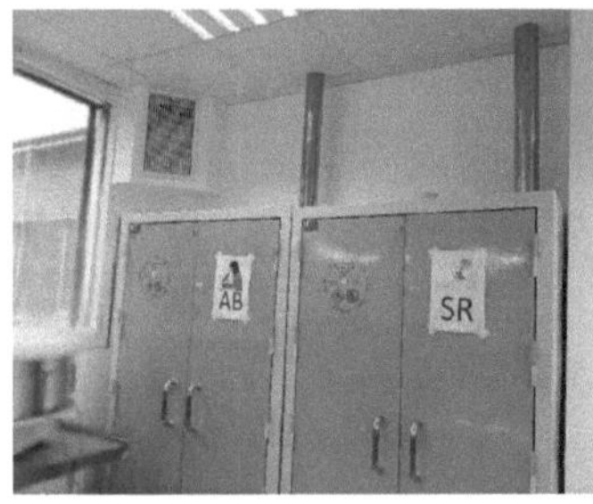

Figure 37: Ventilated cupboards in the macroscopy room

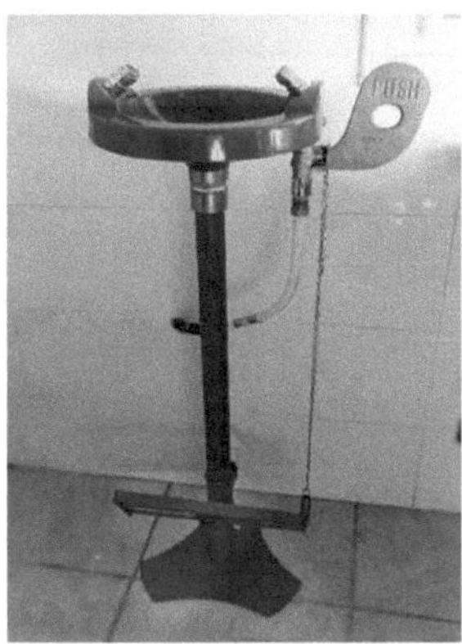

Figure 38: Eyewash device

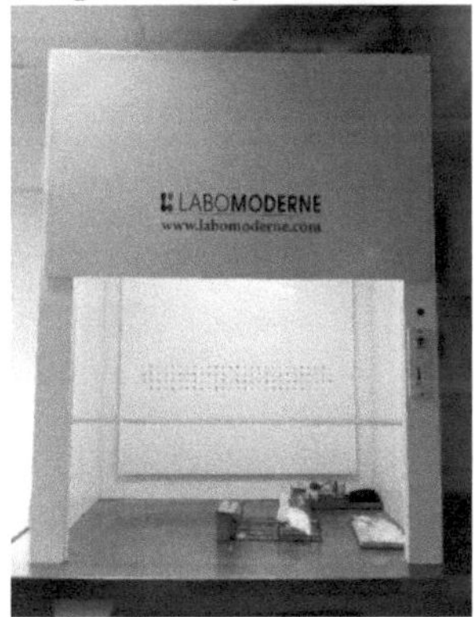

Figure 39: Hood for blade assembly

II.3- Organisational protection measures

The architecture of the laboratory complied with the rules on separation between units. The administrative and office units were separated from the technical rooms, and the reception room was at the entrance to the laboratory and opened onto the macroscopy room. Access to the macroscopy room was indirect (2 doors from the reception room to the macroscopy room or access from the technical room then to the macroscopy room). the staining room to the macroscopy room)Results were delivered in the secretarial unit, which was separate from the technical units. The laboratory was equipped with an alarm system and fire extinguishers. The various waste bags (black, red and yellow) were available, as were the regie boxes and reserve bags. This is shown in the figures below.

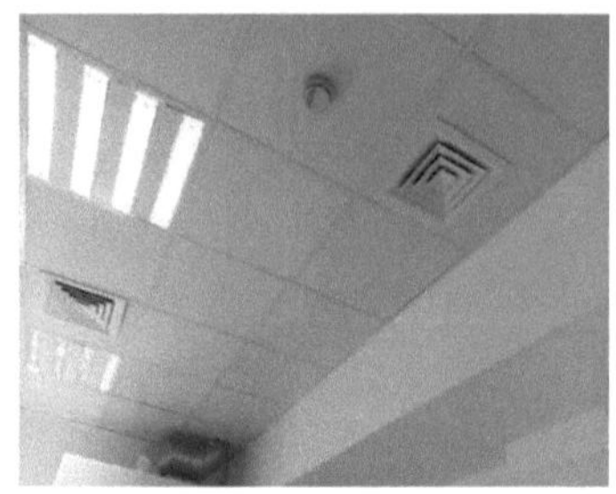

Figure 40: Alarm system

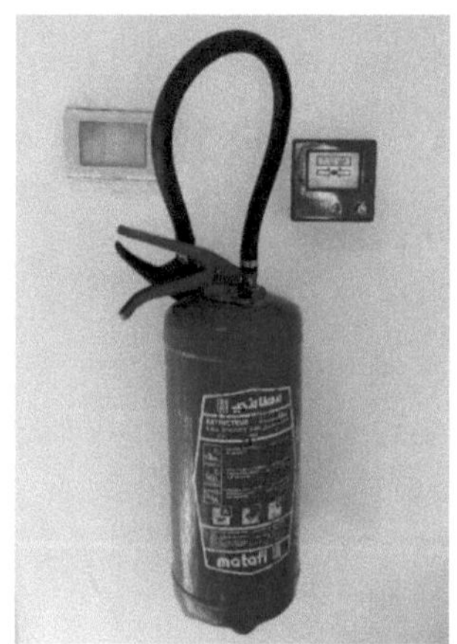

Figure 41: Fire extinguisher in the laboratory

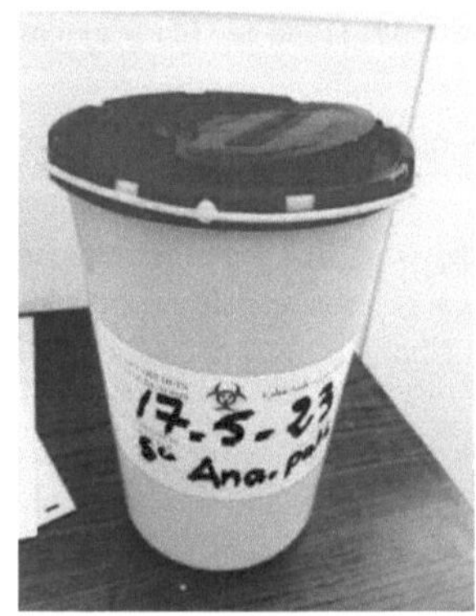

Figure 42: container

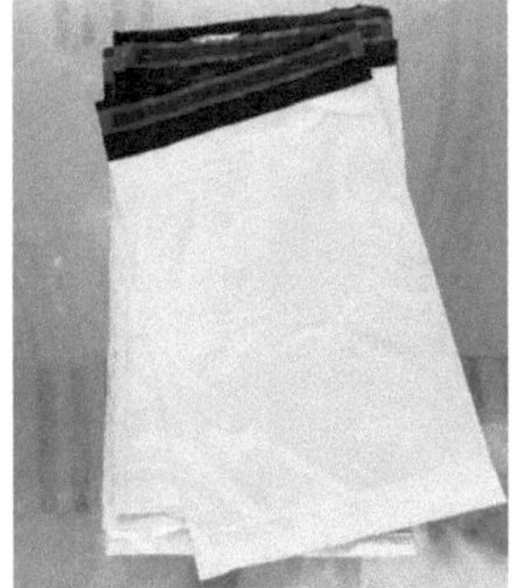

Figure 43: Reserve bags

III. IMPLEMENTATION OF THE 5S METHOD :

To improve biosafety measures, we applied the 5S method, the results of which are illustrated in the following figures.

1 Delete :

Waste and unnecessary objects were eliminated and we obtained a less cluttered bench.

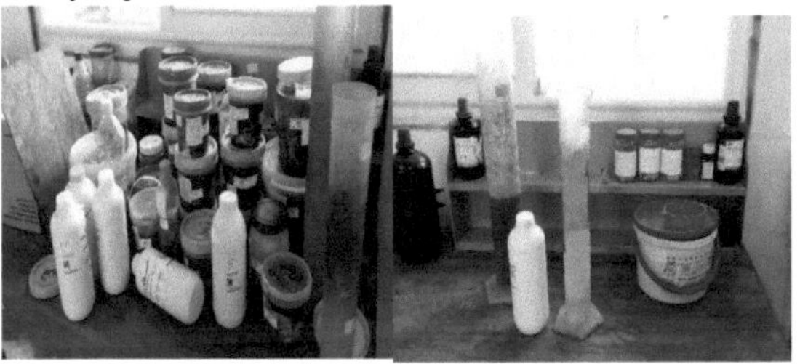

(Before)(After)

Figure 44: Less cluttered bench following application of the 5S method

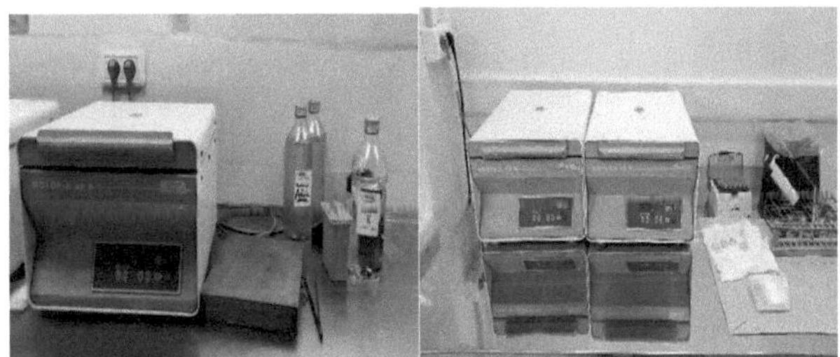

(Before) (After)

Figure 45: Reduced risk of explosion following application of the 5S method

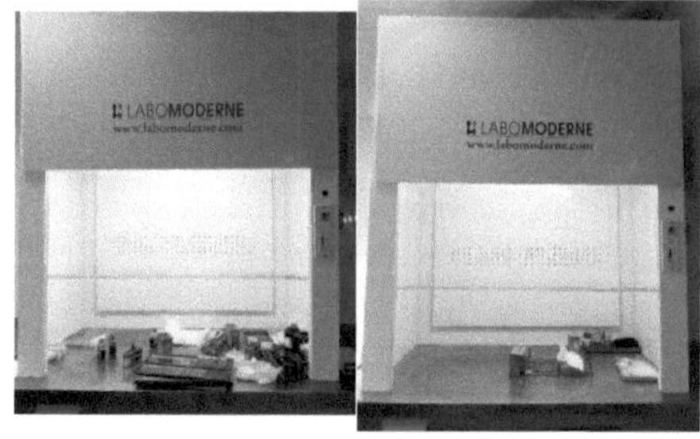

(Before) (After)

Figure 46: Well-organised assembly workstation after application of the 5S method

2 Location :

The equipment was tidy and easy to use, and the risk of injury was minimised by tidying up the dissection equipment.

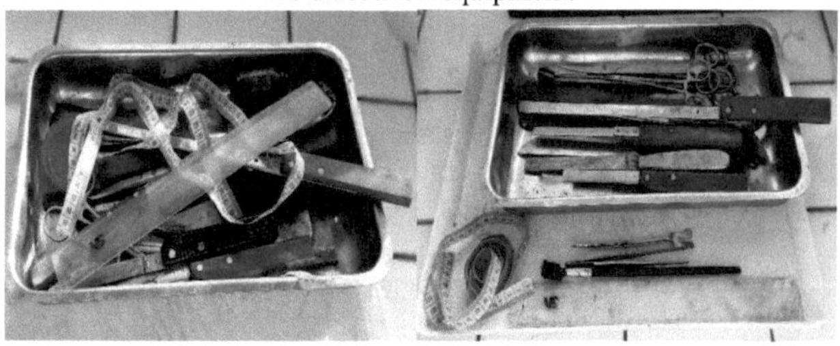

(Before) (After)

Figure 47: Organised dissection equipment

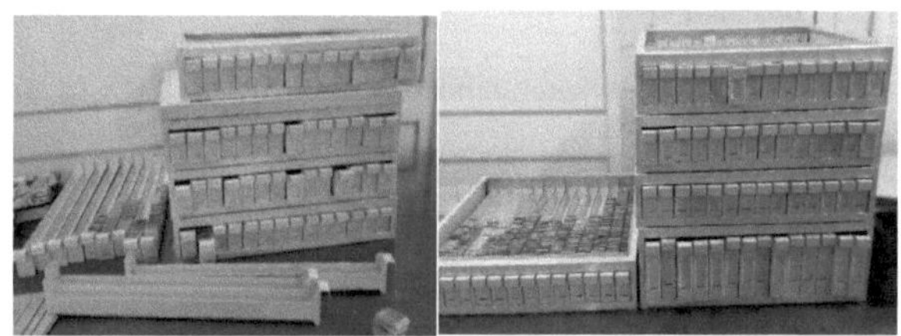

(Before) (After)

Figure 48: Organised block binders

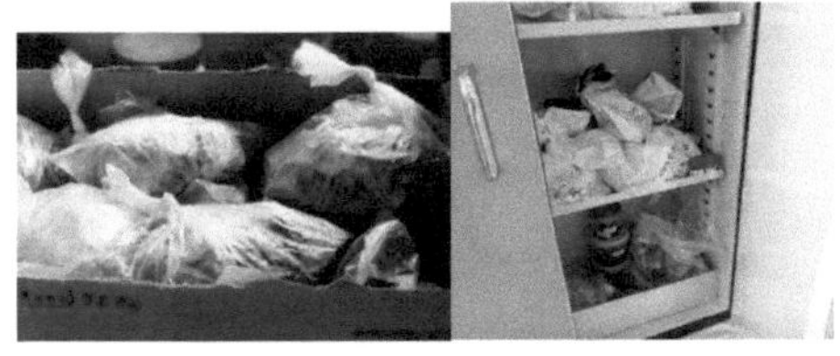

(Before) (After)

Figure 49: Reserves stored in ventilated cupboards

3 Scintillate :

The different units in the laboratory were cleaned and we had a clean working environment.

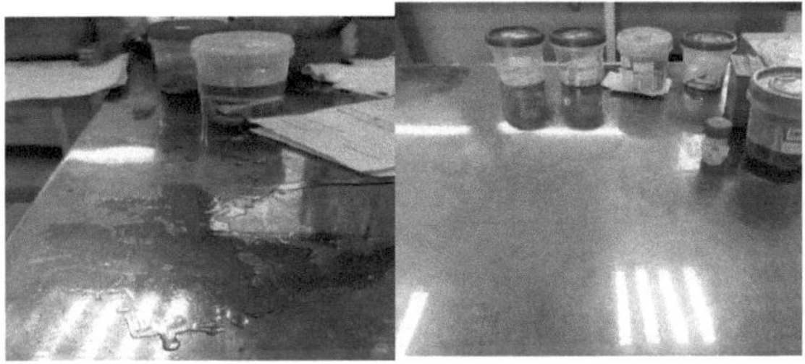

(Before) (After)

Figure 50: Formalin-cleaned workbench

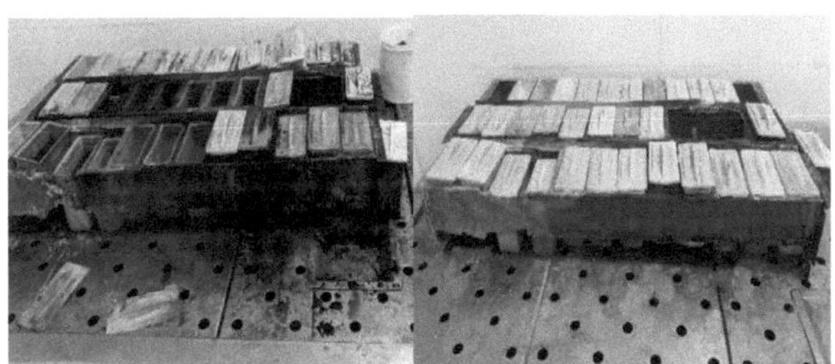

(Before)(After)

Figure 51: Cleaned dye bath

4 Standardise :

Identification posters were affixed to the walls of the various laboratory rooms and brochures were distributed to staff (see appendix). Procedures for risk management and waste management had been drawn up and are now being validated and approved by the hospital's quality unit (see appendix).

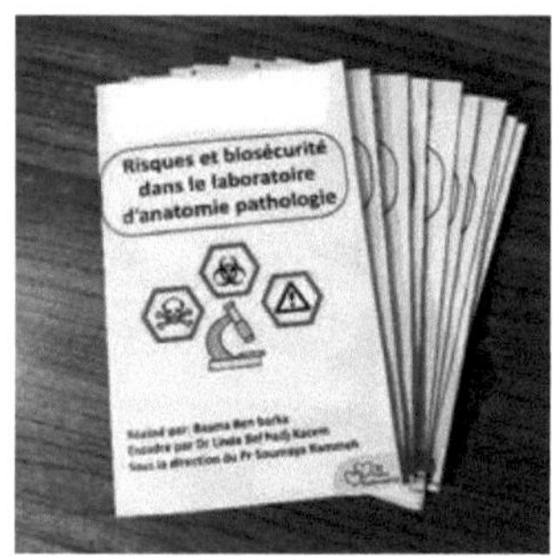

Figure 52: Brochures distributed

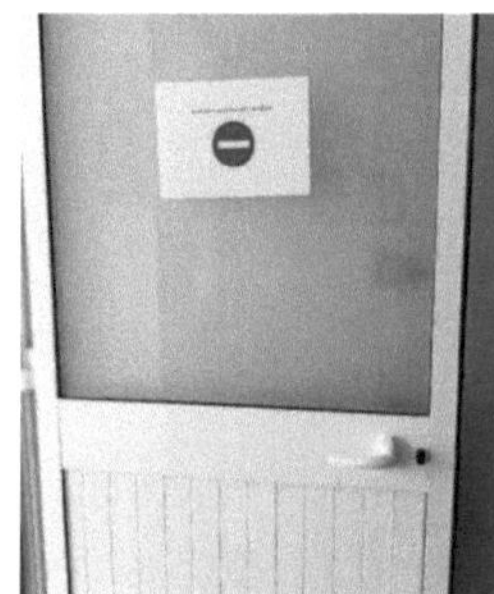

Figure 53: Signage at the entrance to the laboratory's technical rooms

Figure 54: Signage in the technical room

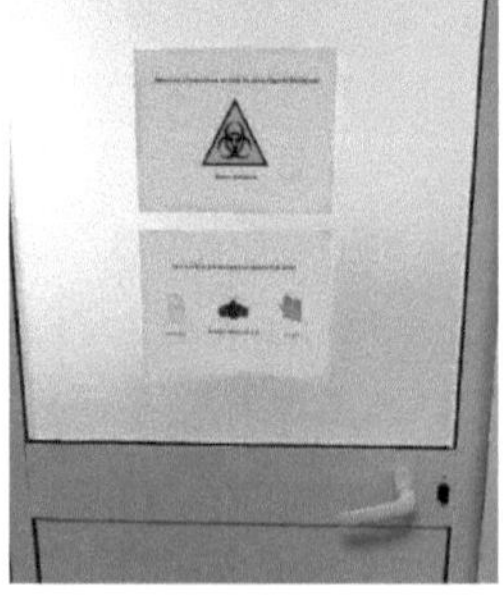

Figure 55: Sign on the door of the macroscopy room

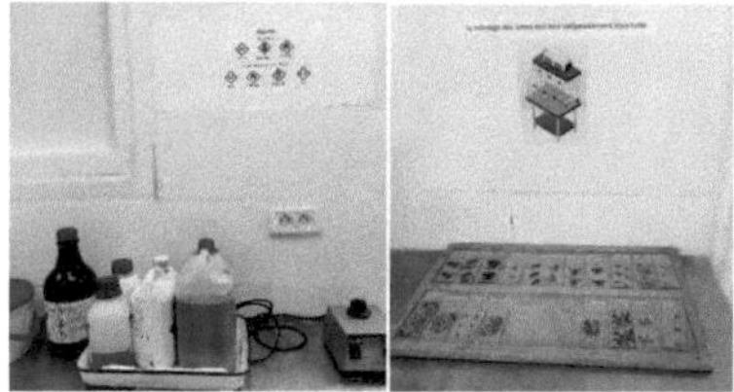

Figure 56: Signs in the staining and assembly room

5 Follow :

The follow-up showed partial compliance with hygiene and biosafety rules.

IV. RESULTS OF THE QUESTIONNAIRE

Twenty copies of our questionnaire were distributed to laboratory staff on 10 May 2023 and 19 copies were handed in on 24 May 2023.

• Participation :

Nineteen responses were collected, with only one staff member not responding to the questionnaire. The participants included : 9 doctors, 7 technicians and 3 secretaries.

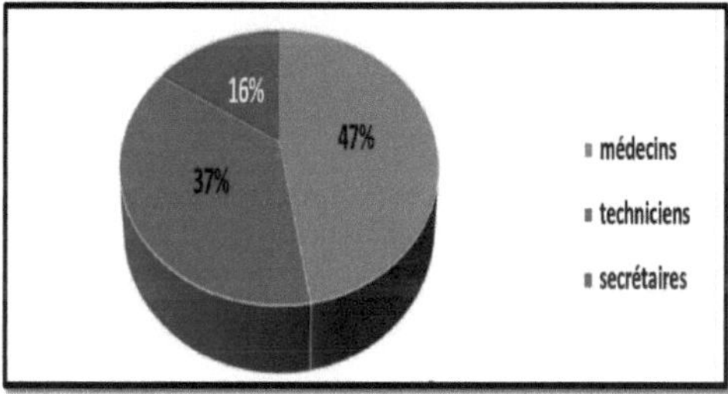

Figure 57: Breakdown of participants

• Length of service in the laboratory :

Seniority in the pathological anatomy and cytology department at the hospital was as follows: Under 5 years: Five participants Between 1 and 5 years: One participant Over 5 years: Thirteen participants

• Assessment of knowledge of types of risk :

For the question assessing knowledge of the different types of risk in the laboratory, 15 participants answered yes and 4 no, including 3 secretaries and one doctor. For those who answered yes, we asked them to name the 3 types of risk. Of the 15 who answered yes, 7 correctly cited types of risk, including 5 doctors and 2 technicians, 5 cited examples of risks and 3 cited a single type of risk (2 cited infectious risk and 1 cited chemical risk).

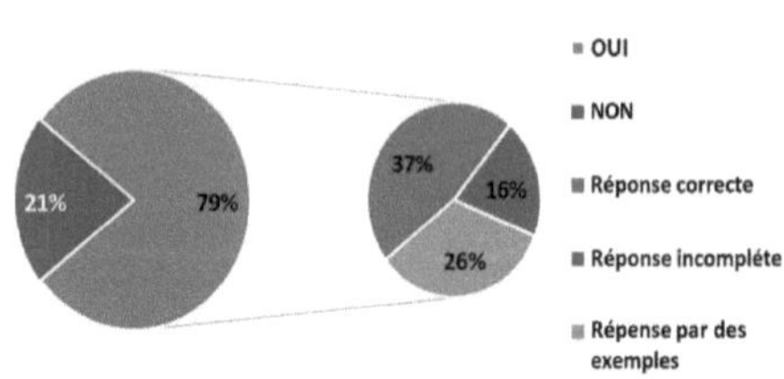

Figure 58: Breakdown of risk awareness responses

- Allergy :

Fourteen participants had developed an allergy since working in the department and 5 answered no. Respiratory allergy was the most common, affecting 9 participants, eye allergy 8 and skin allergy 5. It was noted that 2 participants developed all 3 types of allergy.

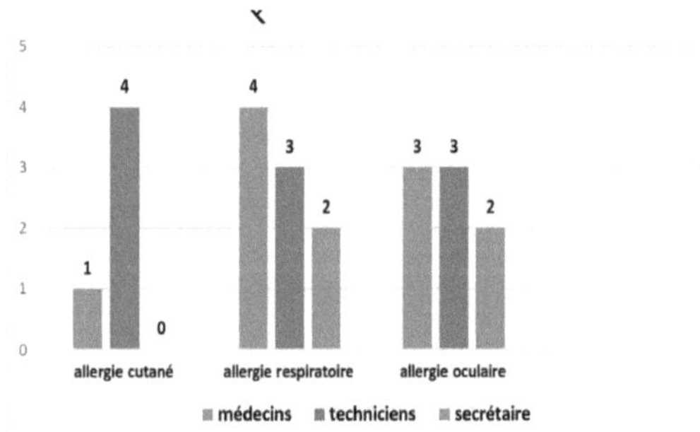

Figure 59: Presentation of allergies according to staff affected

- Musculoskeletal disorders and vision problems:

In this study, 73.6% of employees reported MSD related to their workstation and 52.6% reported vision problems.

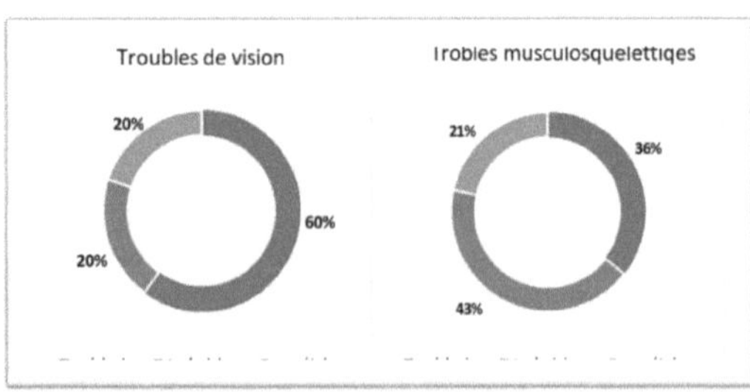

Figure 60: Breakdown of workforce by musculoskeletal disorders and vision disorders

· Chemical risks

The evaluation of the frequency of exposure to chemical risks showed that exposure to chemicals by inhalation was the most frequent, with 15 participants, including all the participating doctors, mentioning that the frequency of exposure was high.
More details on the responses are shown in the following tables:

• Doctor:

Table II: Doctors' responses on chemical risks

	Number of responses			
Frequency of exposure	None	Low	Moderate	High
Cutaneous	2	3	1	3
Lens	0	0	3	6
Inhalation	0	0	0	9

• Technician :

Table III: Technicians' responses on chemical risks

	Number of responses			
Frequency of exposure	None	Low	Moderate	High
Cutaneous	0	1	3	3
Lens	0	1	3	3
Inhalation	0	1	0	6

• Secretaries :

Table IV: Secretaries' responses on chemical risks

	Number of responses			
Frequency of exposure	None	Low	Moderate	High
Cutaneous	2	1	0	0
Lens	1	1	0	1
Inhalation	2	0	1	0

• Physical risks :

The study of the frequency of physical risks showed that this risk is less frequent. Only one participant mentioned that this risk is high and the majority of participants mentioned that the frequency was nil or low.

More details on the responses are shown in the following tables:

- Doctors :

Table V: Doctors' responses on physical risks

	Number of responses			
Frequency	None	Low	Moderate	High
Injury	1	4	4	0
Burn	6	3	0	0
Electric shock	8	1	0	0
Paraffin slip	5	2	2	0
Fire	9	0	0	0

- Technicians :

Table VI: Technicians' responses on physical risks

	Number of responses			
Frequency	None	Low	Moderate	High
Injury	1	3	3	0
Burn	7	0	0	0
Electric shock	6	1	0	0
Paraffin slip	0	3	3	1
Fire	6	1	0	0

- Secretaries :

Table VII: Secretaries' responses on physical risks

	Number of responses			
Frequency	None	Low	Moderate	High
Injury	3	0	0	0
Burn	2	1	0	0
Electric shock	2	0	1	0
Paraffin slip	2	0	0	1
Fire	3	0	0	0

- Biological risks :

Biological risks were common among doctors and secretaries working at reception.

• Doctors :

Table VIII: Doctors' responses on biological risks

	Number of responses			
Frequency	None	Low	Moderate	High
Contact with blood or other biological fluids	0	2	4	3
Contact with loose fabric	0	1	4	4
Contact with leaves soiled with blood or other substances biological fluid	0	3	2	4
Puncture by a used needle	1	4	2	2

• Technicians :

Table IX: Technicians' responses on biological risks

	Number of responses			
Frequency	None	Low	Moderate	High
Contact with blood or other biological fluids	0	1	4	2
Contact with loose fabric	0	2	3	2
Contact with leaves soiled with blood or other substances biological fluid	0	0	3	4
Puncture by a used needle	2	1	4	0

• Secretaries :

Table X: Responses from secretaries on biological risks

	Number of responses			
Frequency	None	Low	Moderate	High
Contact with blood or other biological fluids	2	1	0	0
Contact with loose fabric	3	0	0	0
Contact with leaves soiled with blood or other substances biological fluid	0	0	1	2
Puncture by a used needle	2	1	0	0

• Classification of risks according to frequency of exposure :

The chemical risk was ranked first according to the frequency of exposure, with 73.6% of participants believing that the chemical risk was the most frequent, while 15.7% of participants believed that the biological risk was the most frequent, and the same was true for the physical risk. It was noted that one participant assigned a number 1 for all three types of risk.

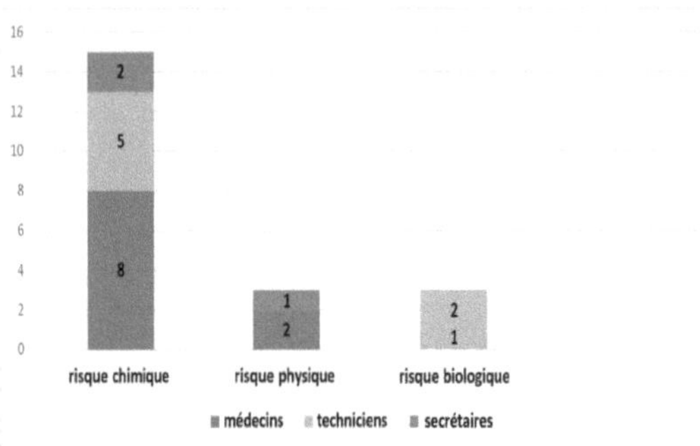

Figure 61: Breakdown of employees according to first-order risk

· Staff training :

Only 15.7% of staff had received biosafety training, including one doctor, one technician and one secretary.

· Staff opinion on biosafety in the laboratory :

The majority of participants thought that biosafety measures in the laboratory ranged from unsatisfactory to satisfactory.

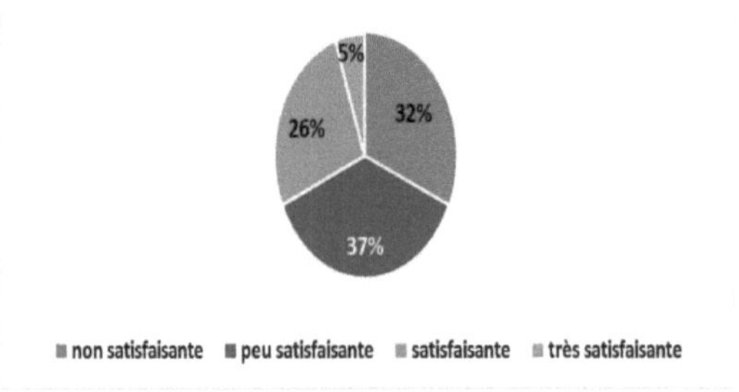

Figure 62: Breakdown of responses on biosafety measures

• Biosafety measures in the laboratory :

The responses showed that 13 out of 19 participants were not aware of the biosafety measures available in the laboratory, and certain individual and collective protection items were mentioned by staff as being absent, such as fire extinguishers, protective goggles and chemical filtration masks, even though these items are actually available. All the participants had mentioned that the first aid kit was not available in the laboratory. Eighty-nine point five percent of the participants had mentioned that cut-resistant gloves and safety signs were missing, as these items are actually not available in the laboratory. Eighty-four percent of staff ticked more than 50% of the biosafety measures listed in the questionnaire as being available in the laboratory.

• Hygiene and cleanliness in the department :

The majority of participants felt that cleanliness and hygiene on the ward was acceptable and none of the staff felt that it was excellent.

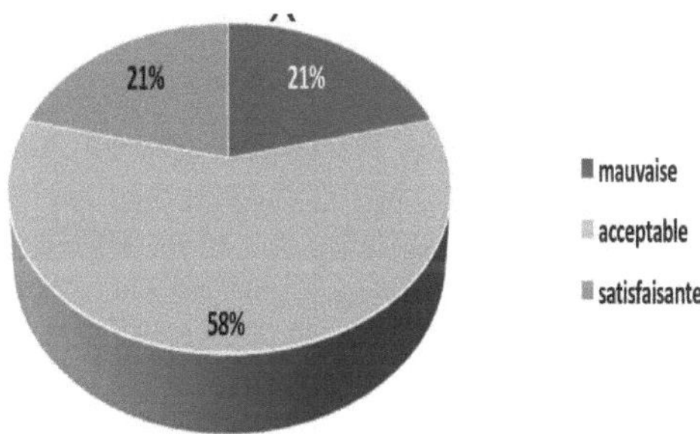

Figure 63: Breakdown of responses on hygiene and cleanliness

Table XI: Summary table of the various risks in the PCR laboratory

Activity	Type of risk	Risk	Cause	Staff presentation	Location exhibition	Corrective action
Receipt of samples	Chemical	Contactin formaldehyde	Poorly sealed container	Agentreception	Hallreception room	Use gloves Containertightly closed
	Organic	Contact with loose tissue or blood	Leaf soiled with blood			Vaccination Secondary packaging, especially for the examination samples extemporaneous

Macroscopy	Chemical	Exposure to formaldehyde by inhalation, skin and eye contact	Extensive use of formalin ventilation Non-compliance with safety biosafety	Doctors Technicians	Room macroscopy	System Ventilation system Use chemical filter mask
	Physics	Injury during tissue dissection	Lack vigilance	Doctors		Use cut-resistant gloves Use scalpel with tip round
	Organic	Contact blood or Fabrics non	Non-compliance with Measures of	Doctors Technicians		Vaccination Work under speaker of
		set by	biosafety			security
		examination extemporaneous				microbiological
Traffic	Chemical	Contact to chemical products when refilling baths the robot	Accidental spillage of chemical products of ventilation	Technician	Room macroscopy	System ventilation system Use gloves, goggles Of protection and mask
Paraffin embedding	Physics	Burn by paraffin liquid	Lack vigilance	Technicians	Technical room	Signage posters for Attention to heat
Microtomy	Physics	Injury when changing blades	Lack vigilance	Technicians	Technical room	Use of cut-resistant gloves
		TMS	Manual activity			Adapt a posture ergonomic
Colour	Chemical	Exposure to dyeing chemicals	Non-compliance with biosafety measures Manual activity	Technicians	Room colouring	Use of gloves, mask, gown and Bezel from protection System of ventilation

Assembly	Chemical	Exposure to xylene and Eukitt	Non-compliance with biosafety measures	Technicians	Room colouring	Work in a chemical fume hood Use gloves, mask And bezel protection
Reading of the blades	Physics	TMS Disorders vision	Use of a long-range microscope term	Doctors	Staff room	Follow the Recommendations the ergonomic posture of The use of microscope
Enter of reports	Physics	TMS Disorder vision	Daily work at the computer	Secretaries	Office secretarial	Adapt a posture ergonomic
	Organic	Contact with blood	Leaf Stained with blood			Use gloves
	Chemical	Contact in formaldehyde	Sheet soiled with formaldehyde			Use gloves
Storage reserve	Chemical	Exposure to formalin	Contact to the attached fabric	Doctors	Room macroscopy	Uses gloves and mask Use appropriate packaging Store in cupboards ventilated
Waste disposal	Chemical	Exposure to chemical waste	Non-compliance with biosafety measures	Workers	All technical units	Use gloves, gown, mask and goggles Tri waste
	Organic	Exposure to unfixed anatomical waste	Non-compliance with biosafety measures			Use of gloves, overcoat, mask and goggles Waste sorting

DISCUSSION

Taking a sample in the PCR laboratory relies on manual techniques, the use of formalin and other chemicals, and the handling of infectious risk agents exposes staff to different types of chemical, physical and biological risks (Ordre professionnel des technologistes médicaux du Québec, 2014). This chronic exposure highlights the importance of biosafety in the laboratory, as well as the implementation of a risk management system to prevent and control risks (WHO, 2006).Our work focuses on assessing the different types of risk as well as biosafety measures in the PCR laboratory at a hospital in Tunis.

This study showed the presence of 3 types of risk in the laboratory with different frequencies depending on the different activities in the laboratory, with technical activities being more risky than other administrative activities.

In the reception room, the receptionist was exposed to chemical risk through contact with formalin via poorly sealed containers or formalin-stained sheets. Biological risk was high when receiving fresh tissues or cytological samples, which may be explained by the poor packaging of the samples (Andrion and Pira, 1994).

Macroscopy was the most exposed activity given the presence of three types of risk: high and chronic exposure to chemicals, particularly formalin, was observed (d'Ettorre et al., 2017). Extemporaneous examination presents a high risk of infection, as fresh tissue may contain transmissible pathogens, exposing the operator to the risk of contamination (Andrion and Pira, 1994). Incidents of injury were also recorded during tissue dissection, due to the force exerted by the manipulator during this precise activity, as well as the use of sharp knives due to the rigidity of certain parts (Fritzsche et al., 2012).

The traffic was automated and, like all automated systems, it can present a risk of leaks and electric shocks, but no incidents were recorded. Inclusion in paraffin was less risky, as liquid paraffin at a temperature of 60°C is fairly tolerable but prolonged exposure can cause burns.
For microtomy, the risk identified was linked to changes in the sharp blades of the microtome; a few incidents of injury were recorded, but the damage was minor.

The chemical risk was frequent in the dyeing activity, which can be explained by the fact that this activity is entirely manual (INRS, 2013).

Assembly is also a high-risk chemical activity, since the slides are immersed in xylene and the Eukitt glue used was toxic (INRS, 2013).

During slide reading, the chemical risk was negligible, while the biological risk was present during reading of fresh cytological fluid slides.

Despite the fact that entering reports is considered an administrative activity, the infectious and chemical risk was justified by the presence of sheets soiled with blood or formalin.

Other risks were identified in connection with the storage and disposal of waste.

We noted the presence of broken blades, exposing grading staff to the risk of injury.
The presence of flammable products near PLCs increases the risk of explosion or fire (INRS, 2013). Reserve storage and waste disposal expose staff to chemical and infectious risks. According to the literature, the presence of these risks is obvious in the PCR laboratory,

particularly the chemical risk, given that the chemicals used are toxic and some of them are carcinogenic (Karami Mosafer et al., 2022) (INRS, 2013).

In addition, there is the risk of infection through the handling of fresh tissues or biological fluids (Fritzsche et al., 2012).Our study showed the unavailability of certain biosafety measures, however ventilation was absent until April 2023 due to electrical works. The absence of ventilation highlights the high concentration and strong odour of formaldehyde in the air.

The installation of the ventilation system improves biosafety at work and increases staff satisfaction.

The personal protective equipment missing was cut-resistant gloves, which explains the repeated incidents of injury (Fritzsche et al., 2012).

Despite the availability of chemical filtration masks, their use was limited, which is in line with the study by Dervaux et al (2020) which showed that only 10% of pathologists used chemical masks.

Gloves were only available in one size (large), so they were not suitable for all staff and this can hinder work.

The architecture of the laboratory complied with standards, although the different units were separated from each other. The reception room was at the entrance to the department and opened onto the macroscopy room, which shortened the path taken by the sample (INRS, 2013). The application of the 5S method in the PCR laboratory helped to improve biosafety measures, in fact this method provided a clean, well-organised and secure workspace by eliminating unnecessary tools that present a source of risk (Drillaud et al., 2016).

The storage of dissection equipment minimised the risk of injury, while the storage of flammable products away from automatic machines or other sources of heat and sparks avoided the risk of explosion.

Cleaning the benches minimised the risk of skin contact with chemicals and blood, thereby minimising chemical and biological risks. In addition, brochures were distributed to laboratory staff to raise awareness of the importance of biosafety in controlling and minimising occupational risks, and posters with information and recommendations were displayed in the various laboratory rooms. In order to gain a better understanding of the risks from the point of view of the personnel exposed and the frequency of exposure, we drew up and distributed a questionnaire. The participation rate was 95%, including 9 doctors, 6 technicians and 4 secretaries; the replies to the questionnaire showed that the laboratory staff are therefore highly exposed to chemicals; 73% of the participants in the questionnaire felt that the chemical risk was the main risk in the laboratory, and the doctors were the most exposed; all the doctors stated that the frequency of exposure to chemicals was high through inhalation.

In terms of allergy, 73% of staff were affected, the main allergy was respiratory, this percentage is higher than that of the study by Fritzsche et al (2012) in Switzerland which showed that 34% of PCR laboratory staff were affected by allergy this can be explained by the strong and chronic inhalation of chemicals in the absence of ventilation system in the previous period in the PCR department as well as the availability of more sophisticated biosafety measures in these developed countries. However, the causal link between the various allergies and work in the laboratory was not well demonstrated.

The other problems identified by the questionnaire were MSDs and vision problems. Indeed, 73% of staff reported MSDs and 53% suffered from vision problems, which is close to the results of Fritzsche et al (2012).

Vision disorders and MSDs were mainly linked to prolonged use of the microscope by the doctor and manual activity with the microtome by the technician (Fritzsche et al. 2012).

In terms of staff training, only 15% of the laboratory's staff had received biosafety training. This percentage remains low compared with the study by Dervaux et al (2020) which showed that around 30% of pathologists had received biosafety training. The lack of staff training explains why some staff were unaware of the three types of risk and why individual biosafety measures were not complied with by some staff, requiring more effort to raise awareness.

According to our questionnaire, only 31% thought that biosafety measures in the laboratory were satisfactory. This percentage is at odds with that of Dervaux et al (2020). This discrepancy may be explained by the lack of financial resources for implementing biosafety measures.

Our study is interesting in terms of its results. It emphasises the importance of risk assessment and is part of the implementation of a risk management system in the ACP laboratory to prevent occupational risks and minimise the risk of their occurrence.

On the other hand, our study was limited in time, as a thorough understanding of the risks requires more assessment time. Otherwise, the assessment of the chemical risks was qualitative, the exposure limit value for formaldehyde was not studied, and the absence of a detector to measure the concentration of formaldehyde in the air made a quantitative study impossible, as did the difficulty of determining the seriousness of each risk.

On the other hand, in our work, the improvement of biosafety measures is based on staff awareness and on the 5S method, given the impossibility of providing biosafety equipment, which is the responsibility of management and is itself limited by a financial budget.

A longer study will therefore enable us to study the causal link between exposure to occupational risks and the development of health problems, and a quantitative study will be more objective in terms of the results obtained.

CONCLUSION AND OUTLOOK

Working in the PCR laboratory exposes professionals to different types of chemical, physical and biological risks (INRS, 2013), this situation encouraged us to assess occupational risks as well as biosafety measures in the PCR laboratory at the hospital in Tunis.

The aim of our descriptive study was to identify the various risks in the laboratory and to evaluate biosafety measures in order to put in place a risk management system to prevent and control risks.Our study reported that the chemical risk was the most frequent, given the chronic and daily inhalation of chemical product vapours; this risk was major in the macroscopy and staining room and not negligible in waste reception and disposal. Biological risks were present in the reception, extemporaneous examination and waste disposal areas, and even in the administrative area, where bloodstained sheets were used; physical risks were minor, and no serious incidents were recorded.

PCR work also exposes staff to MSDs and vision problems, which can be explained by the use of microscopes by pathologists, while manual activity with the microtome was the main cause of MSDs among technicians.

According to our observation, individual (gloves, overblouse, chemical filtration mask, safety goggles) and collective (ventilation system, chemical extraction hood) biosafety measures were available in the department, but cut-resistant gloves, identification posters and a first aid kit were absent. We noted a limited use of personal protective equipment, despite its availability, due to a lack of staff training.

The harmful health effects caused by formalin highlight the need to replace formalin with another fixing agent, but to date no substitute fixative has been able to compete with formalin in terms of quality, speed of penetration and cost-effectiveness. It remains the gold standard with the lowest cost. (Alix, 2010).The impossibility of substitution highlights the importance of improving biosafety measures. A detector that measures the concentration of formaldehyde in the air is desirable for monitoring chemical risks.

Automating manual techniques such as staining and microtomy can be an effective way of limiting damage.On the other hand, external services can play a role in the safety of workers: sampling in a well-sealed bottle and in secondary packaging, as well as a clean request for examination sheet, are crucial to the safety of staff working in the reception area.

The use of a voice recorder at the macroscopy stage and the subsequent drafting of the report protect administrative staff from the risks of contact with sheets soiled with blood or formalin.

In conclusion, the study of occupational risks in the PCR laboratory opens up prospects for the implementation of a risk management strategy specific to the PCR laboratory.

REFERENCES

(Adyanthaya and Jose, 2013): Adyanthaya, S., & Jose, M. (2013). Quality and safety aspects in histopathology laboratory. Journal of oral and maxillofacial pathology: JOMFP, 17(3), 402.

(Alix, 2010): Alix, E. (2010). New fixators in pathological anatomy.

(Andrion and Pira, 1994): Andrion, A., & Pira, E. (1994). What's new in managing health hazards in pathology departments. Pathology-Research and Practice, 190(12), 1214-1223.

(ANGED, 2012): MANUAL FRAMEWORK OF PROCEDURES FOR THE MANAGEMENT OF WASTE FROM HAZARDOUS HEALTH ACTIVITIES in Tunisia 2012

(ASQ, 2009): ASQ(2009)Learning Lean 5S: Quality Pocket Of Knowledge (QPoK)

(Costa et al., 2008): Costa, S., Coelho, P., Costa, C., Silva, S., Mayan, O., Santos, L. S., ... & Teixeira, J.

P. (2008). Genotoxic damage in pathology anatomy laboratory workers exposed to formaldehyde. Toxicology, 252(1-3), 40-48.

(d'Ettorre et al., 2017): d'Ettorre, G., Criscuolo, M., & Mazzotta, M. (2017). Managing formaldehyde indoor pollution in anatomy pathology departments. Work, 56(3), 397-402.

(Dervaux et al., 2020): Dervaux, A., Vaysse, B., Doutrellot-Philippon, C., Couvreur, V., Guilain, N., & Chatelain, D. (2020, January). Occupational risks among pathologists: results of a French survey. In Annales de Pathologie (Vol. 40, No. 1, pp. 2-11). Elsevier Masson.

(Drillaud et al., 2016): N. Drillaud, A. Khalil, C. Siaka, L. Yin: 5S Biologie: un atout pour l'organisation des laboratoires Mastère NQCE, Master QPO Universitéde Technologie de Compiègne, 2015-2016

(Émile et al., 2012): Émile, E., Leteurtre, E., Guyétant, S., Gosselin, B., & Fléjou, J. F. (2012). Pathologie générale. Enseignement thématique. Biopathologie tissulaire.

(Fritzsche et al., 2012): Fritzsche, F. R., Ramach, C., Soldini, D., Caduff, R., Tinguely, M., Cassoly, E.,... & Stewart, A. (2012). Occupational health risks of pathologists-results from a nationwide online questionnaire in Switzerland. BMC public health, 12(1), 1-12.

(Geradus, 2020): Geradus Blokdug (2020), Ishikawa diagram a complete guide 2020 edition

(Harzli, 2021): Harzli, I. (2021). Application to risk management as part of the transition of the quality management system from ISO 17025 v2005 to ISO 17025 v2017: case of MULTILAB laboratory in Tunisia. Journal of Business and Management Sciences, 9(3), 130-144.

(INRS, 2013): Guide pratique de ventilation 22_Laboratoire d'ACP_Version_2013-11-06-07.doc,INRS,2013

(Joshi et al., 2017): Joshi, S., Garg, D., & Jindal, V. (2017) SAFETY MEASURES IN HISTOPATHOLOGY LABORATORY: A.review IDA Ludhiana's Journal - leDentistryVol.1 issue3

(Karami Mosafer et al., 2022): Karami Mosafer, A., Taheri, E., Bahrami, A., Zolhavarieh, S. M., & Assari, M. J. (2022). Comparing formaldehyde risk assessment in histopathology laboratory staff using three methods based on US EPA approaches in the west of Iran. International Journal of Occupational Safety and Ergonomics, 28(2), 1066-1076.

(Lisa, 2017): Lisa Amar Nacache(2017), Assessment of the toxic risks associated with formaldehyde in pathology facilities. Human medicine and pathology. 2017. ffdumas-01669289

(Ordre professionnel des technologistes médicaux du Québec, 2014) : Ordre professionnel des technologistes médicaux du Québec (2014) GUIDE D'ANATOMOPATHOLOGIE

(WHO, 2006): World Health Organization. (2006). Biorisk management:Laboratory biosecurity guidance (No. WHO/CDS/EPR/2006.6). World Health Organization.

Web references

(ISO.org,a): https://www.iso.org/obp/ui/#iso:std:iso:31000:ed-2:v1:fr

(ISO.org,b): https://www.iso.org/obp/ui/#iso:std:iso:35001:ed-1:v1:fr

APPENDIX

Questionnaire

As part of my dissertation project entitled "Risk management and biosafety in a pathological anatomy and cytology laboratory", I am pleased to send you this questionnaire, which consists of 13 questions on 2 pages, with the aim of assessing the different types of risk and biosafety measures in the laboratory.

Please answer these questions NB: anonymous questionnaire

You are:

Doctor technician secretary

Your seniority in the pathological anatomy and cytology department at the hospital is :

Less than 1 year 1 to 5 years more than 5 years

Do you know the 3 types of possible risks in the Anapath laboratory? Yes No

Name them: .

Since working in the department, have you developed an allergy?

Yes skin allergy No Yes respiratory allergy

Yes eye allergy

In relation to your workstation, have you developed:

Musculoskeletal disorders (back, neck, shoulder pain) Vision disorders (short-sightedness, long-sightedness, etc.) No

How often are you exposed to the following chemical hazards: (tick your answer)

*Nil: never experienced

*Moderate: once or twice a month

*low: once or twice a year

*high: at least once a week

NB: same scale for questions 7 and 8

	Frequency	None	Low	Moderate	High
Exhibition to chemical products by	Skin contact				
	Eye contact				
	Inhalation				

How often are you exposed to the following physical hazards: (tick your answer)

Frequency	None	Low	Moderate	High
Injury				
Burn				
Electric shock				
Paraffin slip				
Fire				

How often are you exposed to the following biological (infectious) risks: (tick your answer)

Frequency	None	Low	Moderate	High
Contact with blood or other biological fluids				
Contact with loose fabric				
Contact with leaves soiled with blood or other substances biological fluid				
Puncture by a used needle				

According to your workstation, order the types of risk according to your frequency of exposure: (assign a number from 1 to 3 from the most frequent to the least frequent)
Chemical risks
Physical risks
Biological risks (infectious)
Have you received training regarding biosafety measures in the anapath laboratory :
YesNo
What do you think of the biosafety measures in the laboratory: Unsatisfactory
Unsatisfactory
Satisfactory very satisfactory
Which of the following biosafety measures is/are available': Overblouse gloves goggles Respiratory protection mask cut-resistant gloves Chemical extraction hood ventilation system
Separation between different laboratory unitsfire extinguisher first aid kit posters
What do you think of hygiene and cleanliness in the department :
Poor Acceptable SatisfactoryVery Satisfactory

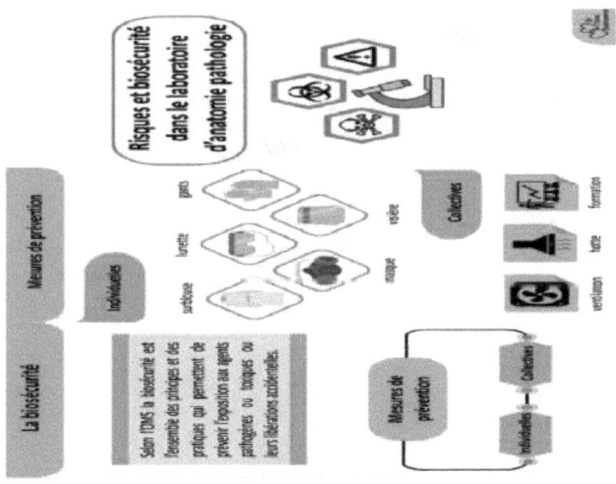

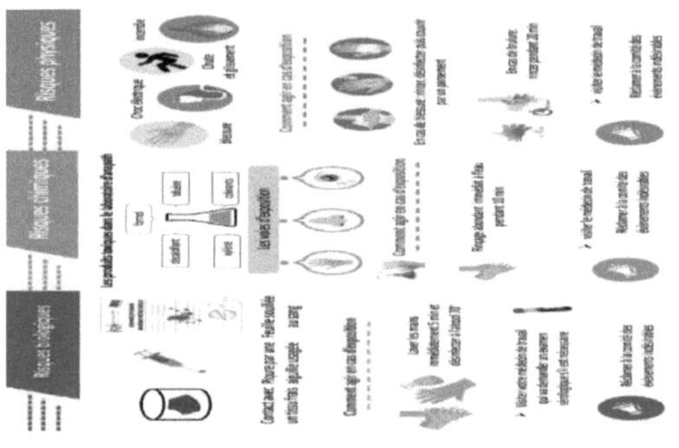

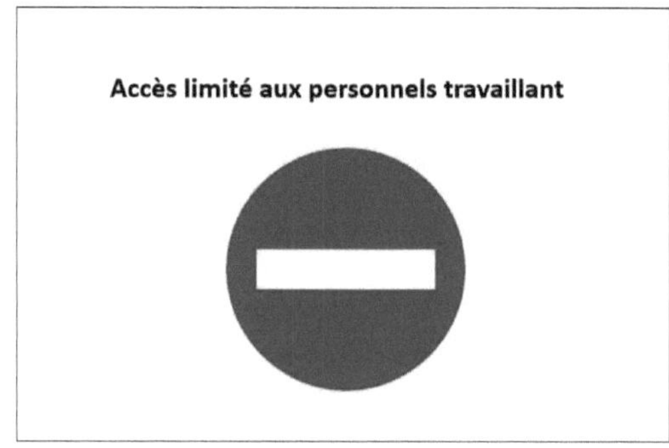

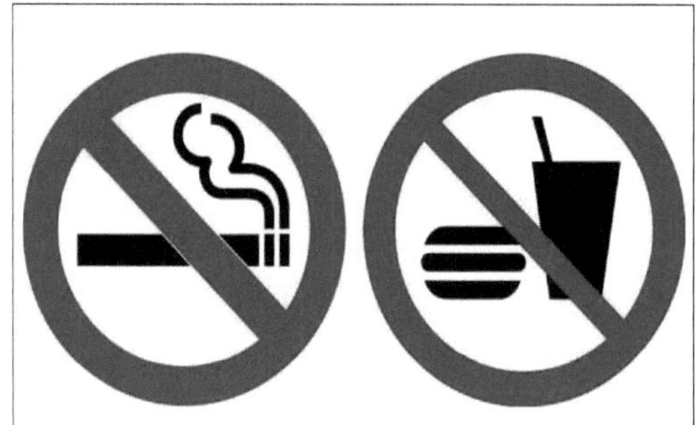

Attention à l'exposition au sang ou autres liquide biologique

Risque biologique

Dans la salle de macroscopie il est obligatoire de porter

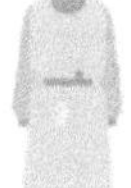

Une surblouse

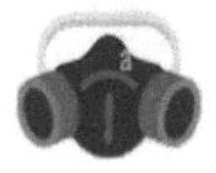

Un masque à filtration chimique

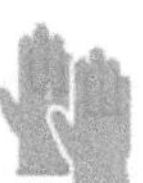

Des gants

Attention

❖ Le formol est :

Toxique

Carcinogène

Inflammable

❖ Le toluène, l'xylène et les décalcifiants sont:

Toxique

Inflammable

Combustible

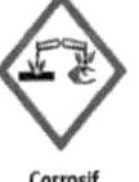

Corrosif

Le montage des lames doit être obligatoirement sous hotte

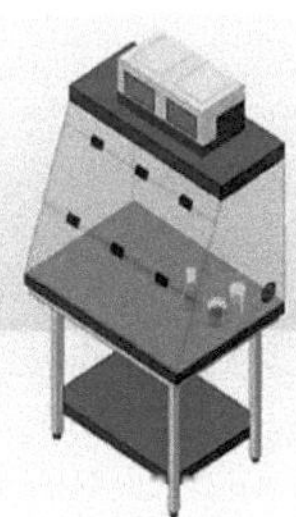

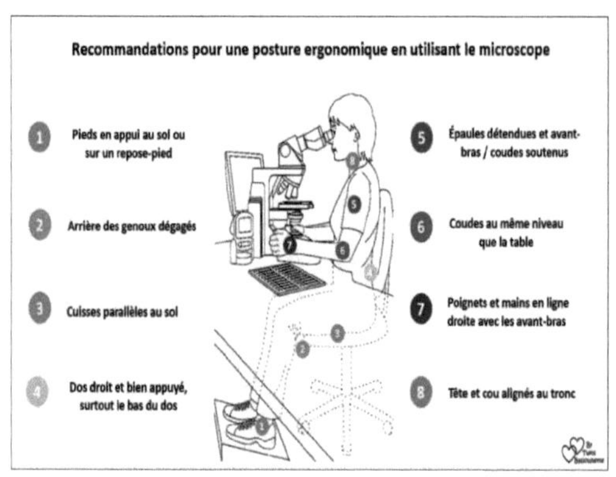
Recommandations pour une posture ergonomique en utilisant le microscope
1 Pieds en appui au sol ou sur un repose-pied
2 Arrière des genoux dégagés
3 Cuisses parallèles au sol
4 Dos droit et bien appuyé, surtout le bas du dos
5 Épaules détendues et avant-bras / coudes soutenus
6 Coudes au même niveau que la table
7 Poignets et mains en ligne droite avec les avant-bras
8 Tête et cou alignés au tronc

SUMMARY

Despite advances in technology, PCR activities rely on manual methods and are characterised by the handling of infectious risk agents and the extensive use of chemicals, which exposes laboratory staff to chemical, biological and physical risks. Within this framework, the aim of our descriptive, observational and prospective study is to determine the various risks in the PCR laboratory and to evaluate the biosafety measures in order to implement corrective and preventive actions. Risk management is carried out according to the risk management process of the ISO 31000 standard by applying the 5M method, which enables risks to be studied, and the 5S method for implementing biosafety measures. Our study reported that the chemical risk was the most frequent, in view of the chronic inhalation of chemical vapours, the biological risk was present in reception and extemporaneous examination, while the physical risk was minor and no serious incident was recorded. According to our observations, biosafety measures were available in the department, with the exception of cut-resistant gloves, identification posters and a first-aid kit.

Key words: *risks, biosafety, pathological anatomy and cytology laboratory*

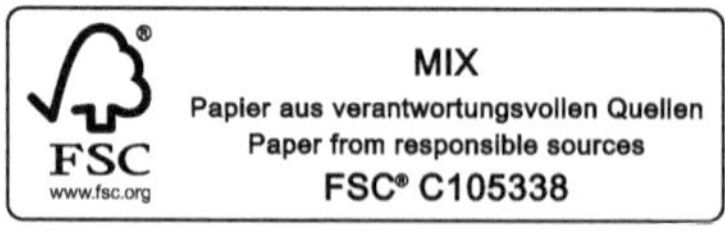

Printed by Books on Demand GmbH, Norderstedt / Germany